Where Soul Meets Matter

Clinical and Social Applications of Jungian Sandplay Therapy

By Eva Pattis Zoja

Translated from German by Benjamin Seaman

Zurich Lecture Series in Analytical Psychology

ISAPZURICH

CHIRON PUBLICATIONS • ASHEVILLE, NORTH CAROLINA

www.ChironPublications.com

Cover illustration by Charles Simonds
Interior design by Danijela Mijailovic
Cover design by Svenia Russov
Printed primarily in the United States of America.

ISBN 978-1-63051-678-9 paperback
ISBN 978-1-63051-679-6 hardcover
ISBN 978-1-63051-680-2 ebook

Library of Congress Cataloging-in-Publication Data

Names: Pattis Zoja, Eva, 1952- author.
Title: Where soul meets matter : clinical and social applications of Jungian sandplay therapy / by Eva Pattis Zoja.
Description: Asheville, N.C. : Chiron Publications, [2018] | Series: Zurich lecture series in analytical psychology | Includes bibliographical references and index.
Identifiers: LCCN 2018049484| ISBN 9781630516789 (pbk. : alk. paper) | ISBN 9781630516796 (hardcover : alk. paper)
Subjects: LCSH: Sandplay--Therapeutic use. | Mind and body therapies.
Classification: LCC RC489.S25 P385 2018 | DDC 616.89/1653--dc23
LC record available at https://lccn.loc.gov/2018049484

Acknowledgments

My thanks go to Murray Stein, who proposed that I write this book for ZLS, showing his great interest throughout the years for our community work.

Without the effort and dedication of my Jungian colleagues, Monica Piñilla, Maria Claudia Munevar, Maria Camila Mora, Ana Deligiannis, John Gosling, Philippa Colonese, Christiane Lutz, Gabriele Mendetzki Mack, Lia Feraren, Cristi Constantinescu, Julia Feordeanu, Delia Descalu, Ema Diaconu, Lavinia Tancusescu and many other volunteer facilitators in eight countries, expressive sandwork would never have reached children in vulnerable situations and changed some of their lives.

My special gratitude goes to all people who have generously allowed me to share their experiences in individual sessions, and who have taught me to be a therapist over many years.

To
Stefano, Sara and Elisabeth
and their playfulness

*"...but often I feel I'm in the role of being
an itinerant bard or shaman."*
(Charles Simonds)

*"I have often encountered motifs which made me think that
the unconscious must be the world of the infinitesimally small."*
(Carl Gustav Jung) [1]

Charles Simonds and his "Dwellings for Little People"

Just as I had finished this present book, a friend of mine, an American art critic who knows my work with children in situations of dire social distress, sent me an interview by Irving Sandler with the New York sculptor Charles Simonds, entitled "Dwelling Munich". It described a social project of his in Munich and there were a few illustrations of Simonds' work. I saw for the first time a photo of one of his "dwellings for little people", dating from the year 1969: small lodgements huddled up against each other, inserted into the recess of a window, and leading a modest but unmistakable life of their own. The buildings, with their windows, doorways and steps formed of tiny bricks, made the concrete ledge

---

[1] (C.G. Jung, C.W. 9/1, & 408)

seem huge and crude. "The little world is the real world!" occurred to me, and I thought of C.G. Jung's description:

"...it seems to me more probable that this liking for diminutives on the one hand and for superlatives – giants, etc. – on the other is connected with the queer uncertainty of spatial and temporal relations in the unconscious. (Jung refers to a Siberian tale in a footnote). *Man's sense of proportion, his rational conception of big and small, is distinctly anthropomorphic, and it loses its validity not only in the realm of physical phenomena but also in those parts of the collective unconscious beyond the range of the specific human. The atman is 'smaller than small and bigger than big',...". (C.G. Jung, C.W, 9/1, & 408).*

For a long time my gaze remained arrested on the little houses, and I devoured the text relating to them. Apparently there existed a world-renowned artist, Charles Simonds, who since the 1970s had been pursuing something similar to what we were: "we" being a group of Jungian psychoanalysts from eight countries who in the last fifteen years had built up a method of Expressive Sandplay for children in vulnerable situations. Time and again we have experienced how highly therapeutic the creativity of children can be if one can provide them with the chance to build a miniature world within a trustworthy environment. And just like Charles Simonds, we too in 2017 had organised a project for refugee families in Munich. The description of his project, "Dwelling Munich", could have been taken word for word from our Sandwork project, and would have applied exactly to the children who had been labelled hyperactive, aggressive, and socially incompetent, and who yet from the very first minute of sandwork had built away at their little worlds with concentration and dedication, and had emerged at the end of the project able to interact with increased calmness, self-assurance, and social skills.

"...and the expressions on these kids' faces are so beautiful because they're engrossed in the kind of wonderland of fantasy, and they're completely candid.

It's as if they are completely relaxed and their faces become themselves in a tender and poignant way. Kids being themselves, you can't help but fall in love with them."

(http://dwellingmunich.de/ausstellung/dwelling-munich/)

It seems that through shaping a little world, the children come directly and instinctively into touch with unconscious energies within and emerge strengthened from the process.

Unconscious, resource-oriented energies appear in the myths and fairy tales of all countries as small, skillful, helpful little people, symbols of one's own creative power, fantasy, and imagination. In the German-speaking parts of Europe there are the "Heinzelmännchen" in the fairy-tales told by the brothers Grimm, and "Erzmännchen" in the Ore Mountains who appeared to miners in distress, and in the regions of the Dolomites dwarves who lived inside the mountains and wrought and forged weapons. Earlier mythological antecedents were the Cabiri (J.W. von Goethe refers to them in Faust II) and the skilled Dactyls of antiquity. It is usually considered great good fortune to encounter these little people; they are generous and helpful but can react with withdrawal and even with revenge if they feel unappreciated, offended, or exploited.

"In the same way the archetype of the wise old man is quite tiny, almost imperceptible..." (C.G. Jung, C.W, 9/1, & 408).

That very night I dreamt about Simonds' little houses, the next day I did research on him, and in the evening tried to make some little bricks out of clay myself to see if they would be suitable for Expressive Sandplay – then I got in touch with Charles Simonds.

Who is Charles Simonds?

Born in 1945 in New York "Charles Simonds is an artist who has been making dwelling places for an imaginary civilisation of little people who are migrating through the streets of cities throughout the world. Each dwelling tells part of the story of the lives of these people, where they have gone, what they do, how they live, and what they believe. Usually passersby, often children, join in as Simonds works and he offers them clay bricks and allows them to add to his dwelling or to make make a fantasy dwelling of their own." *(https://brooklynrail.org/2018/07/art/ CHARLES-SIMONDS-with-Irving-Sandler).*

About how his work began Simonds says:

"At a certain moment I figured out what I was about. I imagined a place; an imaginary place in clay that I put down. I quickly had the idea of an imaginary people. This was 1969 and it was springtime. It was stupid to be doing it inside! I decided to go out to make homes for my little people outside.
(https://brooklynrail.org/2018/07/art/CHARLES-SIMONDS-with-Irving-Sandler).

When it was remarked in a press commentary on his work that the little dwellings are always empty inside, he replied:

"...I'm "inside" each Dwelling as I make it, and imagine it's story. They're really not conceived as small, even though each one is a very small part of an epic story." (https://bombmagazine.org/articles/ charles-simonds/)

As with every work of art, the associations that arise are inexhaustible, scarcely tied to any historical moment in time, universal. One could begin by describing the discrepancy prevailing between the towering skyscrapers of New York and these self-contained circular and spiral shaped miniature structures. Patience and technical ability are a prerequisite for every form of art; in these works, however, a touching solicitude on the part of the artist particularly strikes one as, with the help of tweezers, he builds little brick walls that he glues together. This painstaking procedure of Simonds' has to do with the fact that in his peculiar creative process, apart from himself and the material he's molding, there exists an invisible third component that he patiently and persistently invokes: he can never be certain if the little people will actually come to inhabit these dwellings. Simonds' little people are not individuals but rather social confederacies with a history and a trail of ordeals of their own, epochs of growth and decline. They are peoples who make inventions and can celebrate.

Nevertheless one asks oneself how a grown man, who for all intents and purpose isn't crazy, can stand for days in front of a hole in the wall building tiny houses for imaginary people. The passers-by who gather round him, however, seem to understand what he's doing. One sees on their faces how they inwardly approve: "of course we know this, it's very familiar. We just haven't seen it for a long, long time." And they want to come back and see it again, and recognise it again; and some even want to take it home with them and manage to ruin it as a result. Is this what we call "archetypal"? Simonds' little people are perhaps closely related to invisible buddhistic beings, the "drala's"[2], who assemble wherever good thoughts, good conversation, and lively exchange of ideas flourish amongst humans, and yet who flee at the first onset of friction, conflict, and unrest.

The essential thing about Charles Simonds' work however is that he treats the little people with respect, leaving them alone in

---

[2] *Drala (Wyl. "dgra bla" or "sgra bla") or dralha (Wyl. "dgra lha") — dynamically active non-human beings inhabiting the air element, who are usually invisible to ordinary human perception. As Orgyen Tobgyal Rinpoche makes clear, the inner aspect of drala is connected to the subtle energy system in the body, and the 'secret' aspect to the nature of mind.*

their invisibility. He doesn't want to drag them out into the light or into a museum like the curious shoemaker's wife in the Grimms' fairy-tale did with the elves, when at night she secretly scattered peas on the floor to outwit them into being seen. Unconscious creative energies cannot be directly observed and controlled, one can only create for them a framework. This is precisely what Charles Simonds has been doing now for decades:

"The Dwellings are an incantation of the Little People, as if I'm building them a nest and inviting them to inhabit it. The Little People arrive once the story I've constructed has crystallised enough for them to want to be there. It is also a desperate gesture to give them and me a home." (https://bombmagazine.org/articles/charles-simonds/).

With their close connection to the unconscious, miniature worlds exert an irresistible attraction even to adults, in whom, if they are not in contact with their own creative energy, little worlds awaken strong regressive longings that threaten to drown in malign kitsch. I take "kitsch" to mean any article of cultural heritage that has been torn form its context, thereby being robbed of its ambivalent or threatening aspects. When children on the other hand depict something in a free and protected creative space this is never harmless. In fact it is usually overwhelming, carrying a portion of unpleasant truths, conflict, separation, and death.

Simonds differentiates very distinctly between his own artistic productivity and his socio-pedagogical projects. What the children build is their own art, he stresses. Likewise he has *his* own art and has managed to achieve a degree of acclaim with it. He prefers, however, working "out in the field".

"I'm interested in reaching people who aren't about art, but can think about other things that historically have been the roots of art: beliefs, religion, objects that have a shamanistic power, objects that are interactive, and archetypical narratives. My art is founded by

beliefs; it is the expression of a religion I have invented." (Charles Simonds in: https://brooklynrail.org/2018/07/art/CHARLES-SIMONDS-with-Irving-Sandler).

Here I should like to counter that Simonds may well have invented a language of rituals, but cannot — fortunately enough — have invented a religion.

In his embodiment as sculptor, as therapist, as pedagogue, as storyteller and — as only very few amongst the artists of today — as a modern shaman, Charles Simonds holds together an array of divergent identities. Just how determining an impression can have been made on his art by a holiday encounter in early childhood with the vanished Anasazi culture?

And one cannot stop asking oneself from what source his social vision and his insatiable concern for the creative needs of children may have originated. What role did fantasy play in his upbringing? Charles Simonds' mother, the children's psychoanalyst Anita I. Bell[3], not only made an incomparable contribution to psycho-analysis but also, with keen and sensitive attention, provided for the masculine *and* feminine needs of her sons, which led perhaps to young Charles's being able to remain naturally and continuously in dialogue with an invisible world. And the little people could thus be conveyed safely into the collective consciousness of our times.

---

[3] *In the 1930s Anita I. Bell dared to propound a notion that challenged Freud's theory of castration and at the same time vouchsafed an insight into the development of the masculine identity as seen from the perspective of depth-psychology. She asked herself -- and together with other scientists explored the topic in a research laboratory -- why in the literature of psychoanalysis one has always reflected on only one part of the the male sexual apparatus, namely the penis; whereas the scrotum and testicles, which physically and symbolically stand for the sensibility, creativity and vulnerability of a child and are associated with its anxieties, receive scarcely any notice; are in fact culturally negated. She can experimentally substantiate that unconscious anxieties become noticeable through subjectively non-discernible movements of the scrotum. Her innovative ideas were decades ahead of their time and however effects on a symbolic level not only the individual but the entire patriarchal structure of society. She met with so little response that she resigned from the Freudian Society in New York.*

Table of Contents

Foreword

The theme of this book is the psyche's astonishing capacity and determination to regulate itself by creating images and narratives as soon as a free and protected space for expression is provided. This is true for individuals—children and adults—who struggle with adverse experiences as well as for those who seek a deeper meaning in life. This capacity for psychic self-regulation becomes clearly visible and tangible in the well known therapeutic practice of sandplay.

I will describe two different applications of sandplay that I have developed over the course of two decades. They are oriented towards two different target groups and expand the same basic principles in two different directions.

The first application focuses on individual therapeutic processes based on *kinesthetic imagination*. In this approach, patients are invited to use only sand and water and are instructed to initially disregard verbal narratives and visual imagination, and to concentrate instead on the tactile perceptions of their hands upon touching the sand. These perceptions connect spontaneously with sensorial memories and initiate a process in which attachment models (J. Bowlby) acquired in early childhood constellate in such a clear manner that patients are able to become directly aware of them—it is an immediate, physical experience. The process of kinesthetic imagination is also a creative moment of *new* inner emotional states. I will illustrate this with examples of sandplay processes during which patients engaged with their tactile perceptions and their pre-symbolic and symbolic representations.

The second application is what I call expressive sandwork, which is a method developed especially for children in social crisis situations. This application is practiced today by an international team of Jungian analysts in eight countries. Expressive sandwork takes place in a group setting. Again, the tendency towards psychic self-regulation is central. Using examples, I will show how little therapeutic intervention is needed if the interaction between an adult and a child takes place on a pre-verbal, sometimes even pre-symbolic level, and how a psycho-somatic self-regulation can take charge. I will also describe several expressive sandwork projects in the second part of the book. One such project takes place in Germany in collaboration with the Jung Institute in Stuttgart. It involves working with children of the Yazidi population in Iraq, who have been victims of extreme atrocities by IS and have fled to Germany. Each process illustrates in a deeply moving and convincing manner what a child's psyche is capable of accomplishing even when faced with exceptionally severe trauma. The same is true for children in Ukraine, where Jungian IAAP routers have established expressive sandwork projects in five cities, some of them situated directly in the war zone. The other examples I will describe are from projects in Romania and Colombia.

As mentioned above, these two approaches differ most regarding their target groups; what connects them is a teleological view of psychic phenomena. The teleological point of view means that we consider the aim – in terms of development or relationship – towards which the psychic energy was *actually* oriented when it was obstructed and could not help but produce a symptom. This symptom, however, does the precise opposite and does *not* help reach the original aim. Let us try to illustrate this with an example. If a child has developed a habit of chewing its nails or if an adolescent girl cuts her own skin, a teleological point of view would see this as the best possible means for the child or adolescent to achieve a minimum form of self-efficacy, autonomy, and momentary tension release within their environmental constellation. Both the nail-chewing and self-harm to the liberating point of shedding blood are completely inefficient actions with regard to the unconsciously sought goal of being able to affect something – anything – autonomously. But they are a "better-than-nothing" compromise between the psychic energy driving the child's or adolescent's development onward, like an inner biological clock, and the impeding effect of environmental obstacles standing in the way of this progressive energy. The symptom is more than just a visual expression. It provokes a physical and emotional reaction in anyone who sees the chewed nails or wounds. Chewed nails and wounds "tell" anyone who is perceptive enough to notice that something growth-inhibiting and self-destructive is happening in the everyday life of this child or this adolescent girl. Such implicit "messages" draw reactions of fear, concern, and disgust from the family environment, and they do not help those affected in the least. The symptom serves the purpose of physical tension release, which may protect the patient from organ damage or mental breakdown in the long term, but does not resolve the underlying psycho-somatic imbalance. The psyche and the body will, there-fore, as best they can, continue to search for other more efficient means of expression and for solutions. The psyche and the body never cease to try and counter imbalances. In little children, this process takes place with the utmost intensity, as if controlled by a knowledge that certain developmental steps can only be made at certain ages (Spitz, 1965). The tendency towards psychic self-regulation manifests itself in the ceaseless generation of inner unconscious images. These images reach us adults as nightly dreams and as fantasies. Children have this capacity for psychic self-regulation at their disposal any time and in any place in free, symbolic play. The only precondition is a context free of fear.

"Although play reflects genetically ingrained ludic impulses of the nervous system, it requires the right environment for full expression. ... In most mammals, play emerges initially within the warm and supportive secure base of the home environment, where parental involvement is abundant." (Panksepp 1998, page 281). J. Panksepp showed that even rats immediately and lastingly ceased all play behaviour if just a few cat hairs were placed in their cage (page 18). The moment the motivation system for fear, located in the subcortical structures of the brain, is triggered, the motivation system for play, located in the same area, can no longer be activated. "In all species that had been studied, playfulness is inhibited my motivations such as hunger and negative emotions, including loneliness, anger and fear." (Panksepp 1998, page 18).

We know that learning best occurs in a playful context, and this goes not only for children but adults as well. "It may well be that various neuronal growth factors are recruited during play..." (page 281).

If, in therapy situations, we act on the assumption of self-regulation of the psyche, this means that we, as therapists, do not have to repair a damaged system. Rather, we can rely on this psyche-body-system *itself* always *striving* towards something specific each time anew. The specific something it strives towards? It basically comes down to two main directions: **development** (individuation, in the broadest sense, according to C.G. Jung[4] (1921): and **relationship** (*man is a social being*). Naturally, these two basic human needs are interdependent, and one is not thinkable without the other. During the course of a psycho-therapeutic process, however, they do not occur in a given order. As therapists, we often encounter developmental deficiencies that

---

[4] "In general, it is the process by which individual beings are formed and differentiated [from other human beings]; in particular, it is the development of the psychological individual as a being distinct from the general, collective psychology." C.G. Jung, (1921) *Collected Works*, Princeton University Press, Bollingen Series XX, Vol. 6, par. 757.

deny adults and children the ability to approach other humans emotionally or physically, because they have not found a sufficiently stable relationship with their own inner being. Since they are not yet *on good terms* with themselves, their desire for social exchange with other humans is "on low flame." Even in therapy, such patients are not seeking proximity or even relationship with the therapist. If they are honest with themselves, they actually want to be in analysis and relieved of their symptoms without the presence of another person. A patient once told me, "I would like to speak to you, without you." In sandplay sessions we observe that children with such an avoidant attachment pattern will sometimes play with their backs to the therapist during sandplay or will ignore the therapist throughout an entire session. It is important to them to be able to do this without feeling guilty because it lets them make up for something they presumably lacked in early childhood: playing, undisturbed, in a fantasy world while a caregiver is present and can be called. In concentrating on their inner being in this setting, children need not fear being forgotten by the adult world nor being interrupted by admonitions or instructions. If patients have lacked this both calming and stimulating experience of seeing inner images appear in kaleidoscopic sequences in play or in day-dreaming, the self-regulating tendency of the psyche will immediately use the offer of therapy for that purpose, and the patients will promptly try to discover a new inner state for themselves, in the presence of the therapist. The therapeutic setting is designed accordingly: the patients can, and should, put themselves and their thoughts, emotions, memories, and desires in the centre of focus. The sooner this concentration is focused on the appearing sequences of inner images, and not merely on the conscious wishes, disappointments, and expectations that the patients wish to speak about, the better. Only once a dependable sense of comfort, of being *on good terms with oneself*, sets in can real curiosity for another person arise. In other words, a new relationship model is established. It is the therapist who will likely be tested by the patient as such a first attachment figure who can be approached without fear. During such processes, a medium such as the sandtray offers an unsurpassable therapeutic potential: it is present in the therapeutic setting like a neutral third party, as it were, and allows patients to listen in silence and in their own time to their own body. The body expresses itself over one of its most primitive and, at the same time, sophisticated forms of expression, the sense of touch (we can differentiate an inconceivable number of tactile stimuli with our hands). This sense, in turn, is closely linked to our breathing and to a whole row of further physiological functions, such as heart rate, blood pressure, endocrine function, and hormonal homoeostasis. This is equally valid for children and adults and, therefore, pertains to both of the methods described in this book, *kinesthetic imagination in individual analytic therapy* and *expressive sandwork*. How does this look in practice? I hope I will be able to illustrate that in the following pages.

FIRST CHAPTER

Surprise and Wonder at Oneself

> Since psyche and matter are contained in one and the same world, and moreover are in continuous contact with one another [...], it is not only possible but fairly probable, even, that psyche and matter are two different aspects of one and the same thing. (C.G. Jung *Collected Works*, Vol. 8: 418)

What is the most important experience in sandplay therapy? What is it that draws therapists like us to offer our clients a sandtray against logistical odds such as finding sufficient space in the office for two big boxes and endless shelves of miniatures, having to reorder the miniatures after each session, and permanently having to clean spilt sand off the floor? Sandplay therapists must be especially motivated or particularly fascinated by this method. In my view, there is one great advantage of sandplay compared to other therapeutic approaches. It is the *surprise and wonder at oneself* that often occurs within minutes of having touched the sand. The first touch, in most cases, already induces a sense of wonder: a sensorial perception one did not expect, a state of mind one had forgotten about, a new thought or a movement connected to a visual image. Sometimes the hands move spontaneously, following certain paths, creating openings, finding spaces – "because the sand is so inviting." Sometimes a form unexpectedly takes shape under the hands, as if by itself. – "Oh, how strange!" "I didn't think..." "I've never felt like this – really!" "It reminds me of..." – While the hands explore the sand's consistency, its smoothness, and its readiness to respond to the slightest touch, all sorts of perceptions and emotions go through the clients' state of mind, and they cannot say whether they came from inside or out. It appears to be a circular process, a very subtle but also very persistent and concrete dialogue between the inner and outer worlds, between body and psyche, and more generally, between psyche and matter.

Dora Kalff's Therapeutic Attitude

I remember one of my own sandplay sessions with Dora Kalff in her house in Zollikon. It was the year 1988. Dora Kalff was in her eighties, and she would sometimes doze off while I was working in the sandtray. I was aware of how great a privilege it was to have sessions with this famous therapist of the time, and yet it did not feel that way for me. In fact, I was a little ambivalent about wanting to continue. Since it was quite a trip from Milan to Zürich, I asked Frau Kalff if we could schedule multiple sessions during each weekend, but she did not agree: one session per week would be more than enough, she said. The psyche needs time to process what emerges during the sessions.

In one session, I remember, I had created a landscape without using any miniatures. There was a gentle hill, a river, and a path leading through the image. Once I had created the path, it occurred to me that nobody had ever walked that path, nobody had ever seen this beautiful and calm place before, absolutely nobody. And yet, the more I gazed at the landscape – the precise way the river curved around the hill, that exact view – I realised it was completely familiar to me. It was *my* place. Maybe I had forgotten about it, but there was no doubt that I had known it since forever. And it seemed so clear to me: today I had found it again! I didn't want to leave this session and the sandtray with this unique place that I had rediscovered and created at the same time, a paradox that made perfect sense to me. Such an experience reminds us of what D. Winnicott describes as a transitional object; a child cannot say if it has found the little bear or invented it. There is no distinction, and obviously every creative act is just this: invention *and* discovery.

And then, as though the session had not already been intense enough, Dora Kalff also commented on it. In fact, she used to talk quite a lot during our sessions, not about the work in progress but about other topics. At one point I had taken some sand in my closed hand and had begun to let it trickle gently and very slowly all over this landscape. I was impressed to see how gently this rain fell, and, at the same time, I could feel the tension leaving my body. After a long time of this raining, in which heaven and earth seemed to meet, I heard Dora Kalff's voice: "And each little grain of sand falls into its own place."

It is worth noting that this action – the grains of sand raining from my hand onto this landscape – in Dora Kalff's understanding was not only a representation of nature, such as one might experience water or wind. Through her words, she revealed another symbolic reading with metaphysic consequences. I understood, first through my own somatic perception and secondly through her words, that each little grain of sand did not fall randomly from my hand. In my subjective perception, each grain seemed to *know exactly* where it was *supposed* to fall. This made for a rare and probably archaic experience: that matter had its own purpose (Aristotle) and was animated (animist religions), and that my own action (allowing the rain of sand to fall) was outside *and* inside me at the same time; it was the link between matter and soul.

I once wrote the following in another publication:

> Dora Kalff made concrete use – even nearly concretistic use of Jung's ideas. She wasn't content with imagination, and created conditions, in which unconscious contents can be retrieved from matter itself. In terms of history of consciousness, this counts as a regression. For a concrete object to be charged with psychic substance, for it not to be simply an image of something, but actually to work on its own pars pro toto hearkens back to a very distant phase of human development... Sandplay now gives us the possibility not only of reaching very far back into the individual childhood, but also of a regression to analogous depths in mankind's collective childhood. (Zoja, 2004)

I must point out here that this experience has been the common theme running through all of my work on sandplay therapy in the past 20 years, through my reflections and innovations. It may have been precisely this experience that encouraged me to develop new ways of using this extraordinary tool.

The Third Party in the Room

Thus, in sandplay therapy, we offer the adult patient an activity that requires no technical skills whatsoever. Objections like *"but I'm bad at drawing"* are not even an issue. In the provided three-dimensional space of expression, experiences quickly occur on a number of different levels: tactile perceptions ("...how soft the sand feels..." or "Oh, the sand is cooler than I expected..."), rhythmic elements ("I could keep molding the sand like this for hours..."), haptic experiences ("How good it is to reach deep into the sand, I want to hold it in my clenched hands..."), allegoric descriptions of the state of mind ("My life at the moment is just like this desert here..."), and not least a satisfied desire for beauty ("How wonderful these lines turned out...").

Sandplay therapists do not give directions, nor do they correct or ask "why" questions. They place their trust in the psyche's process of creating images and movement, regardless of whether they believe to understand a meaning or not. Sandplay therapists assume that none of the patients' actions in this search for truthfulness occur by chance. Each gesture, each attempt or hesitation, each correction has an intention – albeit yet unknown. Therapists observe the patient's actions in the sandtray with the same fascination of parents watching their baby's uncoordinated hand movements, wondering *what* it is actually trying to achieve. They have no doubt, however, that it is trying to achieve *something*. At the same time, therapists face inwards and observe changes to their own thoughts, emotions, and body in countertransference reactions to the events unfolding. Somatic forms of countertransference are particularly strong and common during sandplay sessions where only sand and water is used. Therapists enter a psychophysical state of reverie, and their breathing often matches the patient's involuntarily. A very common countertransference reaction is a pleasant feeling of goosebumps running up and down like a warm, tingling rain. In these moments, the therapist's body is surely a resonance box for the energy being released in the patient, just like a guitar string resonating without actually being touched. Asking patients during follow-up about their sensations during those very moments can reveal significant emotional experiences and often syntopic physical perceptions: e.g. patients might describe experiencing goosebumps at the exact same moment.

C. G. Jung (1998) writes in his seminar on Niezstche's Zarathustra[5] from 1934 to 1939:

---

[5] In *Thus spoke Zarathustra*, Nietzsche places special emphasis on the body, especially in *The transmundane* and in *The Despisers of the Body*. In relation to *Self* and the body, the difference between Jung and Nietzsche is that Nietzsche identifies the *Self* with the body, whilst for Jung the *Self* represents both, body and soul.

What is the body for? The body is merely the visibility of the soul, the psyche; and the soul is the psychological experience of the body. So it is one and the same thing. (Jung, 1998, p. 99)

To affirm this, Jung adds:

The difference we make between the psyche and the body is artificial. It is done for the sake of a better understanding. In reality, there is nothing but a living body. That is the fact; and psyche is as much a living body as body is living psyche: it is just the same. (p. 114)

We may ask ourselves why sand is the medium of choice. I have written about this in 2012 and have nothing new to add:

Damp sand enables a wide scope of creative possibilities in three dimensions without any special manual skills being required. Dry sand need be touched only lightly, and already traces are left behind which never seem clumsy or unskilful – even if one draws only a few random lines with one's fingers. The precision with

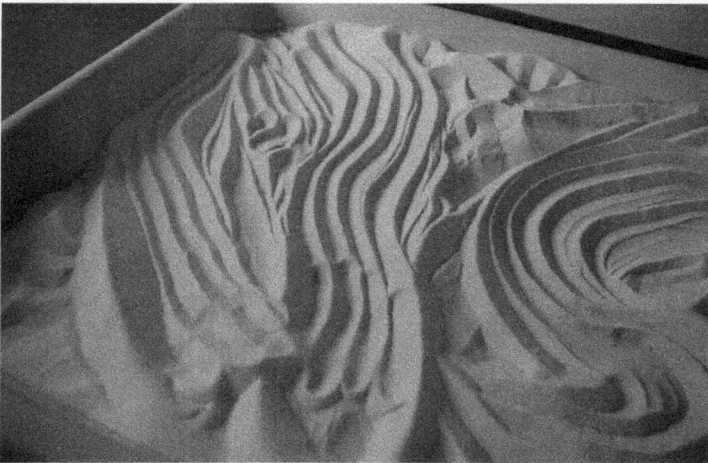

Fig. 1: Traces in the sand

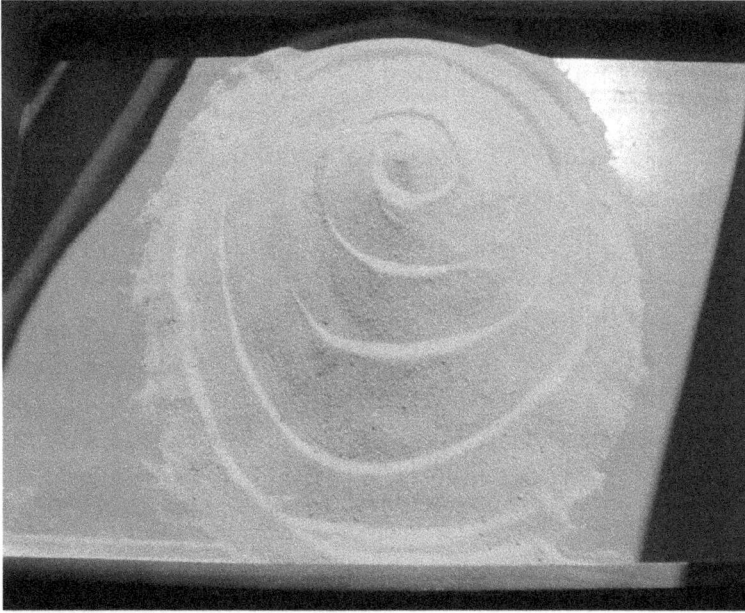

Fig. 2: A three-dimensional spiral

which the grains of sand react to the slightest movement or rearrangement creates an atmosphere of attentiveness. Sand behaves like a very sensitive receiving device that records the slightest influence with total accuracy, as if a million grains of sand were ready and 'listening'. Little by little, sand players' gestures become noticeably in tune with this mood of alertness. [...] Sand formations are easily changed; every destruction automatically leads to new creation. Nothing need be discarded because it is always the same sand, transforming itself over and over again. The sand itself cannot be destroyed, because it already consists of the smallest of particles. (Zoja, 2011, p. 55-56)

The Method's Limitations

Sometimes the mere sight of the sandtray and the therapist's presence are enough to create a hypnoid atmosphere in which unconscious content can become activated. Sometimes, however, such content is activated *too* easily, and we encounter the risks and limitations of this method. I will briefly try to illustrate three situations in which sandplay is not an option because it would likely be harmful for an individual. A patient might give different reasons for not feeling able to use the sand, but all reasons have a self-protective function. All three patients in these examples, two women and a man, had been in analysis for about a year for episodes of depression linked to personality disorders. Each had mentioned on occasion that they would like to try out the sandtray in my therapy room. Once we had agreed on it, the first patient was already quite excited when she arrived for the session. "So today we begin," she said, and her tension was palpable. First, she approached the sandtray, but then she hesitated at a certain distance and appeared to be thinking. I had not yet delivered my words of instruction (which would have begun with telling her she could close her eyes) when she spoke, absent-mindedly: "The sand is so beautiful, so bright and clean. I can't put my sweaty hands in there. I'm afraid I'd make it dirty. I can't. Actually, I don't want this after all."

Something similar happened with the second patient. She had also toyed with the idea of trying the sandtray and the miniatures, but when the day came that we had decided to start, she said she had reconsidered. Unlike the first patient, she didn't make any move towards the sandtray whatsoever. Rather, she turned her back to it and explained that she had thought about how many people had already used the sand, how many bacteria it contained, and the sweat of how many hands... The sand must certainly be very dirty because I, the therapist, couldn't possibly clean it after every session. I confirmed that cleaning the sand involved a lot of work, and that the task was performed at most every six months.

In both cases, the sand in its triangulating presence had fallen victim to strong, yet opposite projections even before the first physical contact. In the first case, the sand became an idealised, unapproachable object, and the patient felt unworthy of its purity. In the second case, it had become an inner persecutor and the patient had to protect herself from its assault and contamination. In the second patient's perception, other people had long since occupied the place she might have wished for, leaving her no possibilities of discovering something of her own there. Early relationship constellations and subsequent behavioural patterns connected to these episodes were plain to see in the life histories and present daily lives of both patients. But they could not be treated with sandplay. Both patients had protected themselves from the consequences of too great an activation of unconscious content. For both, the immediate therapeutic relationship was more important than finding a medium of expression. It is imperative that the therapist listen to these defense mechanisms of the psyche, expressed by the patients in a setting of trust, and respect them without exception.

In the third case, a similar constellation became apparent during the course of two attempts to approach sandplay. This man had been in therapy for two years; he worked in the arts and was hopeful that sandplay might resolve his creative blockade. Sitting in front of the sandtray, he merely moved his hands quickly and skilfully across the surface a couple of times and said, "There – they're sand dunes." In his image, sand was simply sand. No metaphoric or symbolic representation, only literal meaning. Sand is sand. I realised that this would leave almost no room for symbolic expression. We spent the rest of the session speaking about his dreams and didn't touch on the episode again. In the following session, the patient wanted to try again. This time he sat at the sandtray and let the sand run through his fingers for a while. Then he said, "The sand runs through my fingers so easily, and then it's gone. It just vanishes. Nothing remains. No, this isn't for me – this all dissolves and is lost for ever. I'd prefer clay, at least that's

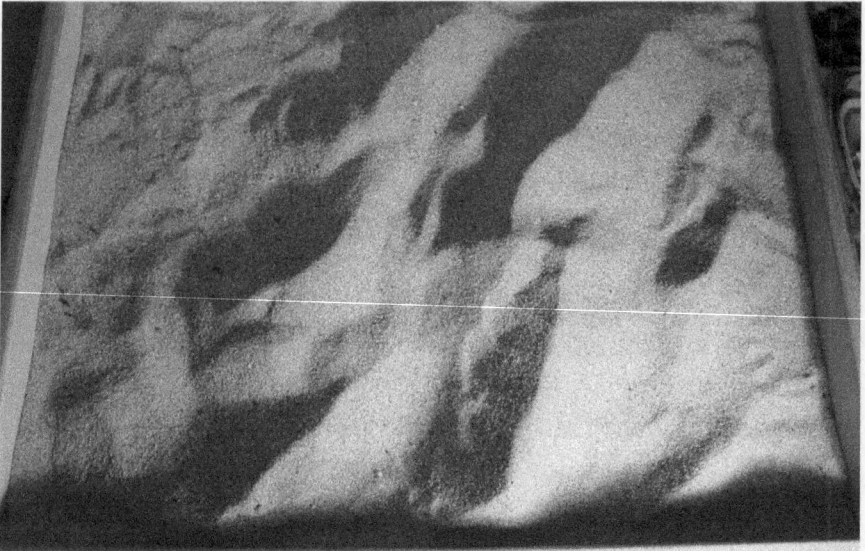

Fig. 3: Sand dunes

something solid to hold." The patient felt clearly that the loose sand would have activated his readiness for dissociation.

Thus, from the very beginning, it is important to understand patients' remarks about the sand, no matter how trivial, as if they were speaking about their inner beings. And it goes without saying that working with the sand is not something that is lightly suggested during the first sessions.

The Opportune Moment for Verbal Exchange

If, on the other hand, a stable setting has been established and if the patient's motivation is firm and leaves enough space for unconscious psychic content, then the first moment of contact with the sand often leads directly to the patient's highly sensitive core emotional issues. The following example should illustrate how important it is that a therapist not comment speculatively on what is being portrayed in the sand. A premature question could disturb a process that takes time to express itself, or it could have a re-traumatising effect. In her first sandplay session – her thirtieth session overall – a fifty-year old woman, whose life history I was largely familiar with, placed both her hands on the sand and remained in that position for a few minutes, attentive to her inner feelings. Then, all of a sudden, her right hand disappeared under the sand and was gone from view, while her other hand remained resting at the surface. It struck me because this disappearing in the sand appeared to be of a different quality compared to a similar behaviour I have observed in many other patients: they appear to bury one or both of their hands in a search for security, as if they wanted to return, unborn, to mother earth's womb and prepare again for the world outside. *This* hand had suddenly dived under and disappeared, and then the left hand began drawing absent-mindedly in the sand, giving me an uneasy feeling. I could see in the patient's expression that something was bothering her, and I asked her how she felt now. She just answered that her hand wanted to stay under the sand. In response, I encouraged her to explore what it was that her hands wanted, and to follow that wish as best possible. Only some weeks later, in a session without sandplay, did the patient return of her own accord to her feelings during that first sandplay session, when her right hand had remained buried in the sand. She explained that her hand had felt dirty and ashamed, that it had felt the need to hide and not be seen. Since we were not at the sandtray this time, I was able to ask if there was a reason for this feeling of shame and dirtiness. With a strong outburst of emotion, the patient began to recount cases of sexual assault by her brother, who had regularly forced her to masturbate him when they were both children. This memory had suddenly surfaced upon her first contact with the sand, and she found it a great relief to be able to bury her hand under the sand. At the same time, she had felt endlessly ashamed.

If traumatic experiences are activated during sandplay by a gesture or movement, these will mostly not be immediately understood by the therapist. Therapists may feel a countertransference emotion or have a hypothesis or question, but will keep all this to themselves for the time being. Depicting an issue in the sand only establishes the preconditions for the issue to be processed on a psychic level. It lifts the issue into the patient's consciousness via kinesthetic perception. Only if the moment for verbal communication is chosen by the patients themselves, can therapists be certain that confronting such an explosive issue will not have a re-traumatising effect. The therapists' task is to process what they see on the outside and what countertransference they feel on the inside, and to reflect on these things for themselves at first. Patients will perceive this psychological digestion on the part of the therapist largely unconsciously, and their psychophysical system will react with further attempts to process the issue at hand. A dream might surface, or further memories, or new somatic symptoms and counter-transference phenomena in the sense of projective identification. Thus, the issue is carried onwards and processed by both parties, each to themselves, until it is ready to be addressed verbally.

Kinesthetic Imagination

When we speak of imagination, we mostly mean images and series of images appearing in front of our inner eye. But imagination can emanate from any one of the five senses[6] and also from kinesthesia, the perception of movement (from the Ancient Greek *kineo* = to move, and *estein* = to perceive). An interesting aspect of sandplay is that an imagination triggered by a movement impulse need not necessarily produce an inner *image* but could lead to another *movement*. Imagination, thereby, remains a physical act and there is a reciprocal interaction between the hands' own movement impulses and the forms they perceive in the sand, which in turn incite new movements, which create new

---

[6] Deligiannis, A. (2012). Cuerpo e Imaginación. Imaginar con el cuerpo en la práctica clínica. Tesis de Maestría en Psicología Analítica Junguiana, Universidad Católica del Uruguay.

forms, etc. The result is a kinesthetic dialogue with the sand. In contrast to Jung's suggested words of direction at the beginning of active imagination ("Think of an image..."), here we wait for an impulse or desire coming directly from the hands themselves upon touching the sand's surface. In a sense, this is similar to the approach of *Authentic Movement* – active imagination through movement (Chodorow 1991) – with the difference that the process in sandplay involves only the hands, and that the patients have not only the therapist's witnessing presence at their disposal, but also the sand's readiness for tactile dialogue. Feeling sand under one's palms is a stimulus that quickly leads to a wide range of sensory experiences. Astonishingly, these experiences are mostly not just problem-oriented, but also resource-oriented. For example, the sand can be perceived by a patient as a dangerous, sucking maelstrom, and then all of a sudden – in the same session and in the same sandtray – as a stable base, as solid, reliable ground. These are embodied, symbolic experiences that have a self-regulating effect on the body and lead the patient's integrated psychophysical system forward to allow a process of maturation. In experiencing the exceptionally sensitive contact with the sand, the patient also experiences the inner and outer worlds as closely interwoven and in constant interaction. This leads to an intense process of differentiating and becoming aware of sensations, feelings, and thoughts. The words used by patients to describe these sensations often sound like variations of Paracelsus' sentence: "As within, so without, as above, so below."

Embodied Symbols

With the following example, I would like to illustrate the holistic effect a symbol can have if it manifests itself not as a visualised imagination, but as a tactile sensation. K., a successful businessman in his sixties and at the peak of his career, was in relationship conflict and questioned his entire life up until that point. He said he saw himself at a crossroads: either to radically change his current life, which consisted largely of a sense of duty and adaptation to the wishes of other people, particularly those of his large family (this was actually what he wished to do, but he was also afraid), or to continue as before because he considered it too late anyway to venture such changes at his age. His manner of establishing relationships with other people swayed between a great desire for autonomy and a strong tendency towards symbiosis, the unconscious desire to become thoroughly dissolved in one's lover. This fluctuation created an explosive mix of guilt and aggression.

When K. laid both his hands on the sand's surface with closed eyes, the first thought that came to his mind and that he uttered was, "I have to tell N. (his extra-marital partner) about this unusual therapy." It was clear to both of us what this meant, because we had already spoken about it: K. lived his own life almost entirely through the eyes and opinions of others. He did not yet have enough inner stability to take his own individual experiences seriously and to enjoy them. They first needed to be confirmed by a counterpart before he could even see them as being real. In short, he largely lived his own life as though seen through the eyes of his partner.

Now K. began to sweep very gently across the sand with closed eyes and remarked that it was a very nice and relaxing feeling. This continued for a few minutes. His movements in the sand could be described as "searching and finding," there was no sense of haste, and I could feel that he trusted the process and agreed with what was taking place in the sand. Then came a moment that tore me from my state of free-floating attentiveness: I was suddenly fully alert because I had heard, almost like an acoustic hallucination, the word "mother," and I could see that the patient had placed both his hands next to each other and had let them sink a little deeper into a depression in the sand just far enough for them to rest there, protected. His facial expression and stance radiated peace and content. After some minutes he opened his eyes and said, "I never would have expected that." He described the feelings that had been triggered by his hands' movements. He had been able to let go and had enjoyed the act of aimlessly creating lines and forms that he could only feel and not see. "Towards the end," he said, "I had the most amazing sensation: I could feel my hands lying in their impressions in the sand. They had found their place, their only possible and true place: inside their own impressions. That feeling alone was wonderful, but when I opened my eyes and could also see how protected my hands looked, it touched me deeply." His depression began to lighten in the following weeks. This symbolic experience of having arrived in his own body's form had been embodied for the patient, had become graphically visible, and verbally comprehensible. I assume that my countertransference reaction was influenced by my theoretical background as a child therapist: it had revealed itself to me in my own imaginative language. The question whether the word "mother" had anything to do with K. himself – for example, whether he had also thought about "mother" in that moment – is not relevant in my opinion. I would consider it a therapeutic misstep to ask such a question. As mentioned before, because we are not only after causal but above all after final explanations, the embodied symbol that K. had experienced on himself was more than enough to take him one step further. Resource orientation is always valuable in therapy, and is naturally effective within any theoretical approach. The approach described here in sandplay can easily be integrated in therapy sessions of other methods. The one condition is that the therapist's respective theoretical approach not be used to comment on the content of sandplay. Even if therapists are accustomed to intervening interpretively during the verbal part of sessions, they must refrain absolutely from doing so during sandplay and must protect the sand images from their interpretation attempts. In the following we will see that, again and again, sandplay reveals its effectiveness in unforeseen ways. It is as if all patients invent, each time anew, their very own way of relating to the sand, which ultimately represents "that which is unknown" to them.

Words of Instruction

From what I have described thus far, it is clear that the words of instruction for such a form of kinesthetic imagination in sandplay cannot be, "Here you can make something in the sand...," just as one would never ask a patient in art therapy to "please draw a picture." Far more, the aim is to help the patient access a hitherto unknown realm of experience, where self-awareness is not the main actor. Therefore, rather than suggesting "to build" or "to create" something, it is best if the therapist encourages the exact opposite: not to create anything, but rather to consider this an exercise to promote the patient's capacity for tactile *perception*. This takes some patience. Since we are used to imagining visually, it will be necessary for the patient to disregard the first ideas and imaginations imposing themselves, and to resist wanting to depict them in the sand. This would likely not produce living symbols, which always have an aspect of unexpected emotional infiltration for both parties. Rather, it would merely translate already-known behavioural patterns into pictorial-metaphoric language, without producing much sense of surprise. In kinesthetic imagination, on the other hand, the aim first and foremost is to perceive senso-motorically what one's hands or fingertips actually *want* when they touch the sand for the first time. And then, in the second instance, to *continue* to focus on the hands' wishes rather than the appearing thoughts and imaginations, as though the hands were autonomous beings with their own intentions, which could also be contrary to the wishes of the patient's own ego. Words of instruction to this effect could be:

If you would like, you can close your eyes and just touch the sand carefully at first. Try to get a sense for how that feels. If you like the feeling, you can lay the palms of your hands on the sand and experience that sensation. Try to feel whether the palms of your hands would like something else or if they are happy to stay like that for a while longer. With your eyes closed, you can tell me any time how you are doing and about any thoughts, feelings, memories, or physical sensations that might appear. Or you can also say nothing during the process, and if you like we can speak about it later. If you have an image in mind or an idea to do or build something specific, it is better to wait a little first and to ask your hands if that is actually what they really want to do. The hands are in charge. Sometimes the hands need a little time to understand this new role, and they would just like to lie there and rest. Sometimes they like to lie a little deeper in the sand, sometimes they would like to make a certain movement. Let everything happen – but every time you feel a new impulse to do something, or see an image that you would like to create in the sand, first take a moment to ask your hands if this is really the very thing that they would like to do right now.

Such words of direction will lead patients directly to their somatic perceptions, and any pressure to need to produce something interesting or beautiful will fall away. This makes way for an imagination that originates in the body itself, and in the most densely innervated part of the body at that: the hands. It is inherent in the suggestion to resist following the pictorial imaginations, to return again and again to the body's perception, that the listening process is slowed down. This intense focus on physical processes relaxes the entire system. Since nothing is expected other than to perceive what is already there, any form of pressure to perform will fall away. Whenever the process or movements appear to falter, the therapist asks, "And what does that hand want now? Is it content? Does it want to stay where it is? Does it feel good as it is? Does it want something else?" After almost twenty years of practice, I have never had a patient experience or do something in the first session that was even remotely similar to the process of another patient. I will try to describe some of the occurring themes in the following chapters.

Photographing Sand Images

The therapist photographs the sand images after each session, but patients cannot take these photos home. This follows the instructions of Dora Kalff (1960), who believed that the creative process continues in the psyche even after a sand image has been completed. It continues to have an effect, in the sense that the image will change and develop in the creator's memory, as is arguably the case with all memories. If the patient were to photograph the image after the session and look at it in the following days, this inner autonomous continuation of the process would be obstructed and the patient's memory would retain the moment captured in the photo. Photographic representation of sandplay processes is a complex issue that has scarcely been studied in the past. I once showed a series of sand images to a wider audience in China. Normally, I only show such images in smaller groups or in a clinical context. I held this talk at a large event on intensive training for volunteers after the earthquake in Sichuan. Since the aim was to inform and train as many people in as little time as possible, I had agreed to also allow outsiders without previous psychological training to attend the talk. I had explained how sandplay could be applied in disaster areas and was showing some photos of sand images and describing the processes by which they had come about, when a man raised his hand and was clearly furious. The translator obviously had great difficulty conveying the man's words, and I am sure that I only heard part of what was said: "It's plain to see that what you've done there is photograph the soul! That is disrespectful. How can you just show that in front of everybody?!" He was beside himself. And I knew that the man was right. I told him so and merely stated in my defense that the listeners present would show the necessary respect, and that my talk was for training purposes. But that was not the point he was trying to make. His argument was that "soul" should not be photographed at all. It is probably no coincidence that this incident occurred in China. It is possible that this ancient culture, where ancestral reverence has played a central role (ancestors as far back as the fifth generation are included in everyday life), is more in touch with soul-related matters and the ways they express themselves. Our western world view seems to be less differentiated in this respect and is, of course, influenced by monotheism; we assume that there is a soul within the body, but we cannot consciously imagine, for example, that this soul could also take the form of a material presence outside of the body. At the same time, however, we value beholding an original masterpiece of art as opposed to an indistinguishable copy, as if we do somehow assume a fresco's colours contain part of the master's soul, which we would like to be touched by.

We handle representations of sand images with the greatest care out of respect for the images' authors. Experience has shown that sand images also always have an effect on the beholders' emotions and influence their psychic state, even (or above all) sand images that would be categorised as unremarkable or neutral on a cognitive level. In my experience, this implicit effect of a photographed sand image on one's emotional state is all the stronger the less cognitive processing occurred during its creation.

In this sense, photographs of sand images cannot be compared with photographs of drawings or paintings. My explanation is that the process of sandplay is able to activate unconscious dynamics much more immediately than drawing or painting. I see two reasons for this: first, sandplay's tactile and kinesthetic nature, and second, because almost no energy is expended on the technical aspects and attention can instead be focussed fully on perception and expression.

SECOND CHAPTER

As Within, So Without, As Above, So Below

In the following, I will try to illustrate how individually patients establish contact with the sand during the first session, and how directly the central issue of their emotional state can be revealed. Patients often recognise these issues as dominant patterns of experience and behaviour, as a kind of leitmotif in their life that repeatedly asserts itself despite their conscious intent. The symbolic forms of expression described in the following examples are the result of a kinesthetic sensorial perception which is surely developed *before* our capacity for pictorial imagination, during the first months of life, when, we assume, infants still experience the outer world as indistinguishable from their inner worlds. Even scientists attempting to descriptively approach these psychic realms, which are so inaccessible to consciousness, choose the poetic form, such as Daniel N. Stern (1990) did in his *Diary of a baby*. The words of an actual poet are much more immediate. Adalbert Stifter (1867) remembers "dark spots within himself,": „Es waren dunkle Flecken in mir. Die Erinnerung sagte mir später, dass es Wälder gewesen sind, die ausserhalb mir waren" (Stifter, 1867), which he only later understood to be "the forests outside me." At this point, I would like to emphasise that my therapeutic approach is indeed based on the foundations of development psychology, but that I do not express this approach and, as I have mentioned, do not communicate it to the patient as a suggested interpretation. It is a way to categorise the patient's life history for myself, but it goes without saying that it is just *one* approach and by no means the only one. Each point of view bares the risk of forcing incomprehensible phenomena into specific patterns, thereby reducing them instead of enriching them with context. In this case, it would mean regarding the patient predominantly as a helpless infant, which would naturally have a disastrous influence. It is not just the last decades of scientific results in attachment theory, with confirmation from neurobiology, that make me personally adhere to my point of view of developmental psychology. It is a far simpler observation: patients are able to access their inner selves through sandplay *despite* my psycho-developmental approach and are able to take on their current life situations and effect real change. In other words: as long as a therapist doesn't mistake theoretical background for objective truth, it will not disturb the patient's self-exploration and will grant the psyche a maximum of space in which to unfold its tendency towards self-regulation by means of symbolic content. Thus, I ask the reader of the following examples not to be distracted by the psycho-developmental approach because the described process of realisation by sensorial perception, the fascinating *sensorial hermeneutics*, is by no means tied to this approach. It is no more than a pair of glasses that benefits my own desire for cognitive understanding, but it becomes less and less important as the process unfolds. Take the following example: a patient builds a compact form in the sand during a session or multiple sessions. Let us assume it is a hill. This three-dimensional, tangible and palpable object clearly makes the patient content, proud, and happy. During the following sessions, two of these forms take shape, and it becomes ever clearer that the two hills are connected and in relation to one another. Again, the patient is clearly satisfied and even moved by the objects. After further experimenting, three such forms take shape under the patient's hands. The presence of this third hill plainly relativises the two others. I read this sequence as a representation of the early childhood experience of unitary reality (Neumann, 2014), which, once consolidated, leads to the experience of "me and you" (the mother figure or primary caregiver) and then to a further level that transcends and triangulates this primary relationship (the father figure or society). Not only is a new element added in each phase, but each new element shakes up what had been there previously. Child, mother, father. Or, in abstract terms, from one, to two, to three. In sandplay processes revolving around individuation processes, we often find analogies to alchemical processes described by C.G. Jung (1953). In the continuation of our example this would be the transition from three to four, which represents a reorientation of psychic energies (C.G. Jung on Quaternio and the number eight as the double Quaternio), and then the appearance of the number five (quintessence as a paradigm that incorporates the previous levels and carries them one further). Thus, psycho-developmental and archetypal approaches are reciprocal and are conducive to capturing the therapist's interest and fascination, leaving no space for reductive interpretations that might dismiss a phenomenon as "...nothing but..."

Pausing, Resting, and Making Space

When invited to touch the sand and to ascertain what their hands would really like, many patients lay their palms on the sand, listen for a while, and then discover that their hands would actually like to stay just as they are. To rest and to do nothing. The hands might let themselves sink a little deeper into the sand, coming to rest inside the depression they created, and patients' expressions will relax and they will breathe deeply. Others feel an urge to make more space for themselves after their first contact with the sand. The damp, heavy sand in front of them suits this urge perfectly, and so it is pushed away with great satisfaction until the light blue base of the sandtray appears. This gesture is liberating and is often repeated numerous times.

A., a woman in her forties, closed her eyes, laid the palms of her hands on the sand, and waited for a feeling or an impulse which, as mentioned above, was to come not from her imagination but from her hands themselves. After listening intently for such an impulse for a while, she said, "There is so much energy in my hands. They really feel as if they are full of energy." I remembered a dream A. had told me about, in which she discovered new, previously unknown rooms in her apartment. She continued, "It's as if all of this energy were flowing down to earth. It starts here in my heart, then flows down both arms into my hands and then into the earth." There was a clear hint of uncertainty in her expression, so I asked her, "And how do you like that feeling?"

"I don't really know. Somehow the energy is being wasted – it's flowing into the earth and nobody is using it. *I* don't even know what I could do with it," she said. I didn't comment on this, because it would likely have led to conscious reflection and distracted from her sensorial perceptions. A. began to sweep gently across the sand's surface, exploring its expanse. She described how limitless and vast the sandtray appeared to her. "There is so much space here. And even more space!" She said that it wasn't easy to reach the upper limit of the sandtray because it was so far away from her. A. felt along the upper edges of the sandtray, her eyes still closed. "This border gives me a sense of security and support because there is so much space inside of it. I can scarcely believe I have all this space for myself!" Her palms glided across the wide expanse, deep breaths accompanying her movements. Under her sweeping movements, the sandtray appeared expansive and generous, even to me. "I feel light as a feather," A. continued. Having grown up in confined, middle-class conservative circumstances and in a psychopathological family constellation, and suffering from psychosomatic ailments (mainly gastro-intenstinal problems), it must have felt incredibly liberating for her to have this vast potential psychic space at her disposal. A. opened her eyes and her elated sense of wonder turned to disappointment: "Oh, the sandtray is that small!?" It was as if the sandtray had shrunk and now struck her as confined and unattractive. She closed her eyes again, to return (successfully) to her previous impression. Then she opened them once more to see the space shrink anew. Next, she concentrated on trying to reconcile these two conflicting impressions by alternately closing and opening her eyes while exploring the expanse of the sandtray with her hands. It became clear that A.'s tactile, kinesthetic perception was resource-oriented (a new potential habitat was there to be explored), while her visual sense alone perceived the sandtray as a metaphor for the confines of her daily routines. It is safe to assume that the offer to create something in the sand would not have opened such an immediate path to A.'s psychic potential, had her tactile sense not been allowed to take the lead. A. quite simply would not have been able to *see* the sandtray's "astonishing" expanse, while her tactile perception, which came before the visual sense in evolutionary terms, led her spontaneously to this self-regulating inner realm where something new could be created.

Towards the end of the session, A. concentated once more on the energy she had felt in her hands, arms, and upper body, and which had now, she explained, spread to her head. "It is as if this energy was all around me, even above me." After the session, while saying goodbye, she beamed and said, "I feel like a new person."

After having successfully accessed this source of psychic energy within herself thanks to her tactile sense, A. now began to think about how she could use this new force at her disposal (energy and space) in her daily life. In one of the following therapy sessions she spoke about how the sandtray's narrowness she had perceived with open eyes could represent her conscious attitudes and habits from which she had been trying to break free for so long. I, for my part, could confirm to her that her vitality, her fantasies, and creativity had been hemmed in by her intense fears and her guilt towards her

45

demanding family. The expansive, almost limitless space she had perceived with her tactile sense represented her life still largely unlived, which she was in the act of exploring through therapy.

What distinguishes sandplay as a method in this case, and in many others, is the patient's sense of surprise and amazement at herself, which had constellated very quickly and was accompanied by strong emotions. It was not the therapist who had pointed out to the patient that two contradictory modes of behaviour were at loggerheads with one another; the patient had experienced this without the therapist's help, and she was impressed with the coherence and assertiveness with which her own psychophysical system had expressed itself. This not only gave her faith in the therapeutic process. Above all, it instilled confidence in her own psychic process, which had demonstrated such autonomy and creativity. I would like to emphasise again that psychic self-regulation occurring through free creativity in a protected space does not merely portray a current outer or inner conflict (it is not merely problem-oriented), it *also* always presents possible ways out of the conflict. It does this by uncovering resources that were already present dormantly and may have just been "waiting" to be linked to self-awareness in order to unfold their full development-stimulating effect. A. experienced her innate tendency towards psychic self-regulation in the here and now, and she did so through her own body. She had not just *spoken about* something in therapy, things had *actually moved* thanks to an energy *from within herself*. All of these processes quickly helped her take concrete steps to change her life situation. In the following months, A. bought an apartment in a part of town that did not match her bourgeois background and habits, but where she felt comfortable. She decorated the apartment according to her own taste – again, breaking with her family of origin – her social relationships changed, and she received a lot more recognition at work because she no longer hid her talents. In short, the space and the excess energy she had found in sandplay became embodied symbols of an actual, concrete space she could claim and develop in her life. At the same time, she could feel her abdomen relaxing and her breathing becoming deeper during the sessions. The entire process was accompanied by dreams, one of which I would like to recount here. A. was sitting in her father's car. She was steering the car, and it was immensely difficult to do so because she was sitting on the back seat with her own steering wheel, while the front seat was empty. The absurdity of the situation hadn't occurred to her in her dream. Remembering this image proved helpful throughout her therapy to heighten her awareness for situations in daily life where she risked exhausting herself by making decisions "from the back seat."

Between Heaven and Earth

O. reached into the sandtray and buried her hands in the damp sand. She enjoyed the feeling of not having to do anything in particular and felt at ease. After a while she began to push the heavy mass of sand away from her, thus creating space for herself in the lower part of the sandtray. Then she brought all of the sand back to her end of the sandtray, only to relish pushing it away once more. It felt like an immense relief and she repeated the movement a few times, clearly enjoying it. "I made room for myself – I'm finally making space for myself," she said later, when I asked her how she had felt. "It was so liberating!" This act of making space for herself, which she repeated similarly over a number of sessions, corresponded with a newly discovered desire to say "no" to the many obligations in life she didn't want. She began to realise how little space in life she actually claimed for herself due to her insecurities and her drive for perfectionism. O. was the daughter of an immigrant family. All of their lives, her parents had taken pains to adjust to their host country, trying to be as inconspicuous as possible and standing out only through their sense of duty and work ethic. As a culmination at the end of this process of pushing-

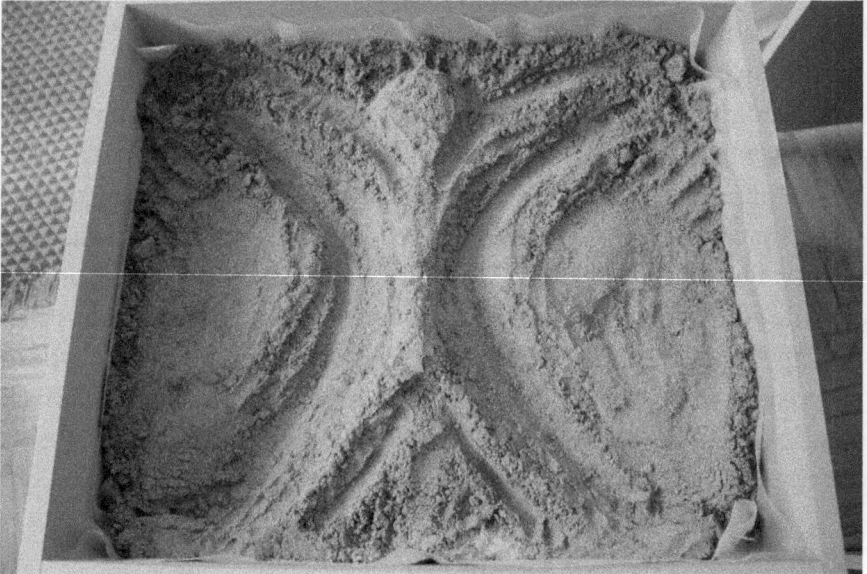

Fig. 4: Between heaven and earth

away and creating space, O. made the following image that clearly filled her with great satisfaction. (Fig. 4) She commented, unprompted, that this figure reminded her of Leonardo da Vinci's Vitruvian Man, creating space for himself between heaven and earth.

A Conflict of Hands

With her eyes closed, the first contact with the sand puzzled S. She was surprised how asymmetric her two hands felt as they lay before her on the sand. While her right hand could barely contain its desire for movement and action, her left hand lay in the sand like a dry leaf and couldn't be moved from the spot. S. found the sensation so unpleasant that she tried something else. She took some dry sand in her closed hands and let a thin trickle of sand fall from each one, as if they were hourglasses. She repeated this action a few times. A look of displeasure soon crossed her face. She bemoaned how unevenly the sand trickled from her hands. The sand flowed as it liked from her left hand, far too quickly in her mind, while her right hand was able to control the flow of the sand and let it trickle just as she wanted it. The two mounds forming under each hand even looked completely different. The mound under her right hand looked alive, while the one under her left looked like it was made of wasted or dead sand that was good for nothing. The asymmetry had cropped up again. No matter how hard she tried, S. was not able to get both hands to match each other. Intense, conflicting emotions accompanied each of these movements. The right hand was afraid to let too much sand trickle out, while the left hand relished its own extravagance. In one of the following conversations, S. compared this unresolvable conflict with two contradictory habits that were making her life difficult. Either she was strict with herself, dieted, worked excessively, and demanded perfection in her actions, or she had phases of self-indulgence, when she would eat vast quantities of chocolate, not even get dressed in the morning, and spent the day watching television. This process repeated itself a number of times over the following sessions, until S. suddenly had a playful inspiration and crossed her arms. "I've tricked them!", she called out excitedly. "Now it will work!" And lo and behold, with her arms crossed, both hands were able to let the sand trickle down in equal measure. The body had found a solution that would not have occurred to her mind. It seems reasonable to see the trickling sand as a representation of her psychic energy, its aim being to achieve better economic equilibrium between a number of opposites, between the inner and outer world, between giving and taking, and between omnipotence and impotence.

The Sound of Sand

V. was a psychologist in training who rushed (so she said of herself) from one appointment to another and couldn't really wind down for weeks on end. In her first sandplay session she began circling her hands rhythmically in the sand, both in the same direction and then in opposite directions. As she did this, the friction of the grains of sand on the base of the sandtray made a fine, steady whooshing noise. "It's like the sea," she said and listened intently as if the sound were coming from elsewhere. "And like the wind...I could listen to it for hours. It actually gives me goosebumps." Occasionally she turned her hands over, to see how it felt to stroke across the sand with the backs of her hands. This conveyed an impression of great intimacy. The atmosphere became calmer and more concentrated. Next, V. began to feel through the sand with her finger tips and picked tiny grains out of the sand – "seeds", as she called them. She held one of these little grains in her fingers, her eyes still closed, as if she wanted to explore its tiny dimensions. It was an infinitely delicate and subtle act. "Even such a tiny grain has its own consistency," she said, and she laid the seed aside. Then she started circling her hands again, her rhythm accelerating until it began to feel hectic. At the same time, the sandtray struck me as being limitless, as if it had no border. The sand's surface appeared open and exposed, without a protective container around it. I felt an impulse to contain V. and protect her. Knowing her biography, I saw a parallel with a state of great psychological vulnerability that had shaped her childhood. She had grown up in a family clan that lived off organised crime. The female members, in particular, were not able to develop any self-worth other than through illegal activities, which always involved fear of the police and of being arrested. Towards the end of the session, V. again picked out individual grains of sand and placed them on a little pile in the middle of the sandtray. "One mustn't underestimate them, even if they're still so small," she said, smiling. The session ended with a sense of satisfaction for V. She wondered at her own ability to achieve mental and physical equilibrium.

A Lack of Depth I

D. was a retired industrial sales representative with a decades-old addiction problem. After his first contact with the sand, he thought there was far too little sand available. He had buried his fingers a little way into the sand and had already reached the base. "I would so like to get to the bottom of things," he said, "but I am also so afraid of doing so. I am afraid there might be no depth in me. That is my greatest fear, that there is nothing there to get to the bottom of. I think that is why I drink." As we know, it is risky to try to establish a causal relationship between an addictive behaviour and an external situation (because my partner..., because my employer..., etc.). Discovering a causal relationship with an *inner* situation also carries a certain risk, unless the individual is fully aware that every persistent addictive behaviour develops a psychophysical momentum, and that the putative causal relationships might only serve to sustain it. On the other hand, it is remarkable in this case that the patient was confronted with an important existential question through his contact with the sand and that he was able to relate it with his problem by himself. Though there was no constellation of a visible resource in this case, there was a lowering of defences and a willingness to face an inner problem.

A Lack of Depth II

After a two-year analytical process involving sandplay, M. experienced a "lack of depth" in the sand in her last session rather than her first. We had already looked back on all of her sand images together, which was very moving for M. She was impressed by her own vitality and creativity that were apparent in the sand images. She proposed making one more sand image, not least because she wanted to understand if she did indeed want to bring the process to a final close. In this session, she made an unexpected discovery: there was far too little sand in the sandtray and she couldn't dig down deep enough. "One reaches the base right away," she said, disappointed and puzzled at the same time because she had never noticed this before. "But today I would like to dig down deeper." After a number of frustrating attempts to reach the desired depth by pushing the sand together to form a mound and digging down in the middle, she eventually found a satisfying solution: she made a hole in the mound and placed a mirror in its centre. Looking in from above, something glinted mysteriously at the bottom, as though infinitely distant. She was content – she had created depth where depth had been lacking before.

"But I was there..."

When G., a young woman, decided to first make contact with the sand, her immediate reaction was: "The sand is so cold!" There was a note of reproach in her voice, but she did not remove her hand from the sand's surface. After a few moments' silence, G. said, "I just had a funny idea. I was wondering if you would like to join me?" She knew that this was not intended as part of the process, and she didn't actually wish it to happen, she was merely surprised at the idea. Then a sentence burst from her, "But I don't want to play alone!" And with it came a strong emotion and childhood memory. She was sitting with a little shovel and bucket on a wide, empty beach and there was nobody there – no adult far and wide, just endless grey sand. G. cried while recounting this story. There was no need to ascertain whether this was a real childhood memory or a representation of an emotional state. After a long silence, her hands anchored tightly in the sand, G. said, "But *I* was there. I know that now. *I* existed, even if nobody else was there. *I* was there!" The painful memory of past neglect, which had already announced itself at the beginning of the session in her perception of the "cold" sand, was emotionally endured and was enriched by a new element of consciousness: the perception of her own, autonomous existence. Thus, a possible solution had surfaced along with the problem. It was easy to see resource-oriented psychological processing at work here. It is remarkable that G.'s primary focus wasn't on the former lack of caring adults, but rather on the former child itself and on the acknowledgement of its existence despite its abandonment. This new, inner tenderness towards herself or, in other words, this constellation of a positive mother archetype, had played out successfully in the first twenty minutes of a sandplay session. For G., this also shed new light on her past relationships that were characterised by dependence, fear of abandonment, and submissiveness, patterns that she was able to identify and work on in therapy.

A Demonic Presence

B. suffered from asthma attacks and depressed moods. She was a writer, but she regularly felt obstructed in her creativity. She was prepared to examine her "deeper problems," as she called them, with the help of sandplay. She was about to reach into the sand in the first session, when she paused and spoke after a moment's deliberation, "It's as if someone inside me had said, '*Are you honestly going to start playing now? That's the last thing you need in your already precarious profession. It's childish! Do something useful with your life for a change.*'" I asked her if there was a figure that went with the voice, to which she answered that it was the voice of her father, who was hyper-critical of everything she had ever pursued and who was clearly trying to mess up yet another one of her plans. I reflected on the fact that such an inner voice might actually not be entirely wrong with regard to B.'s life history. She had initiated but then abandoned a lot of activities, she had little professional and emotional stability, and she repeatedly overextended herself. An inner, positive authority focused on reality could surely prove useful, but it could not be incorporated in so destructive a form. Since her father's voice was apparently preventing her from claiming the sand for herself, I asked B. if she would like to portray the voice in the sand. This was a concrete suggestion on my part, and the mere fact that I had uttered it should have been a warning to me because I don't actually find concrete suggestions useful. With swift movements, B. created a face in the damp sand, which protruded from the middle of the sandtray like a relief, the mouth grim and the eyes blank and staring. B. found the face unpleasant and, as if banishing an evil ghost, she drew a large X over the place where the neck would have begun if the sand face had had one. I thought of B.'s asthma. And about the fact that we know this behaviour (vehemently crossing out something with an X) from children's drawings, where it is understood as a desperate attempt to make traumatic experiences undone. B. had drawn the X with her finger so deeply that the light blue base of the sandtray became visible. The fact that the X had no physicality compared to the face therefore gave the crossing out gesture an impression of helplessness and desperation. Nevertheless, B. said that the voice had now stopped reprimanding her. We continued the rest of the session in conversation. In the following session, B. selected dry sand and wanted to use the miniature figures, but she said that she didn't really know what to make. After some deliberation, she decided to illustrate a dream that had frightened her. In the dream, a woman (she chose a Native American Indian woman for her sand image) was threatened by a man (she chose a man with a raised axe).

Contrary to our original plans and supposedly due to external circumstances, B. was not able to continue her therapy. I can't say whether this termination was related to the constellation of a negative father complex, either synchronistically or fatefully. It certainly gave me food for thought in retrospect that neither of her sand images had shown any visible activation of inner resources. It is safe to assume that working with the sand was not the right choice for B., but I had not understood that at the time.

So Gentle...

N., a woman in her forties, had built a life for herself far away from her dysfunctional family of origin but found herself in a conflictual relationship and had great difficulty establishing her professional life. A common theme in her dreams was that her dream-self disappeared. It dissolved like a mist or was invisible. In her first contact with the sand she stroked delicately over the surface, then laid her hands on it and said, "It's so gentle. I hadn't expected that. How can sand be so gentle?" Then she curled her fingers a little, forming a hollow below her hand, and let her hand sink into the sand so that the cavity was now filled by a little mound of sand that had formed under her hand. N.'s facial expression showed she was content and relaxed. "It's nice how the sand takes shape under my hand. It's my own form – it's just right. It's like a miracle that I can rest my hand on this exact form, my form. She remained like this for a while, fascinated by what she was experiencing. When I saw that she had become a little uncertain, I asked what I always do in moments like this: "What would your hands most like to do now?" "They would like the space below them to always be completely filled. No empty space, absolutely full. There should always be something as solid under them as now," she responded. There followed a series of deep breaths, and she noticed them as well. "My breathing reacts as soon as I feel that firmness beneath me. I can stay here. Just stay here," she continued, concentrating on her perceptions. After a long pause, N. began to run her hands very lightly over the sand's surface. I was fascinated by the sensitivity of the gesture. She was clearly in the process of discovering something new for herself. "I can't believe how gentle the sand is. And that this is *me*... I'm always so hard and tense." Tears came to her eyes. "I never thought that life could be so gentle! I think I have been waiting for this for 45 years without knowing it was possible."

Having assured herself of a solid inner basis, N. was able to respond to her hardness (also in the physical sense of a muscle carapace, protecting her from overly intense emotions): she could allow herself to connect with – literally to touch – her own sensitivity, and she was deeply moved by the experience. It was as if she had discovered, in the archaeology of her soul, an unexplored area which had been there all along. Such a paradox situation is typical of the appearance of living symbols.

In the second session one week later, the preceding processes were consolidated and expanded by one new element: delight in playing. First, N. noticed that her upper body and back relaxed as soon as she touched the sand. After rediscovering the "solidity" under her hands she said, "Now my hands would like something new." She took a little sand in her fingers and let it trickle down. "How lovely! It was solid and full last time, but how it can change! It is still full, but also light and gentle. I can play with it; it is constantly changing. I can do what I like. Now it is like baking pudding or kneading dough, or I can pat across it with the backs of my hands. Now it is gentle again, it makes me sad. There is a great sadness that goes with such gentleness in the world. And yet, *everything is connected with everything else.*" She was astounded by this last remark.

In a further session a few months later, in a depressed mood, N. went one step further. She began the session reluctantly and unenthusiastic about the sandtray. "I'm tired. I'm out of strength and I don't know what there is left to discover in the sand." I noticed that N. neither lay her hands on the sand, nor reached into it. I wondered if she was trying to avoid too strong an emotional involvement and was afraid of being overwhelmed by her own sadness. But I had greatly underestimated N.'s psyche's tendency towards self-regulation. N. took a tiny bit of sand between her fingers and said, "These tiny grains calm me." Then she assured herself of the experiences she had made so far: her hands sought out the solid forms under their arched palms and she spoke of emptiness and fullness. Then she said, "It feels good. I always have something solid in my hands here. I never come away empty-handed. And it isn't as tiring as I had thought at first, it is so calming. And, actually, all it takes is a single tiny grain, a single one..." She held a grain of sand between her thumb and index finger and regarded it for a long time (although it wasn't even visible) and said, "*Yes, all it takes is a single grain of sand and you are no longer alone!*" She had to laugh at her own remark. "Yes, it's true, the smallest fraction of an amount of something is enough!" In my understanding, it was a first, tentative experience of a stable presence outside of herself: a first representation of "you." Thus, the foundation for a new readiness for inner and outer dialogue had been laid. N. left the session reassured, calmly cheerful, and grateful.

Daydreams Protect Against Loneliness

Sometimes the surface of the sand is stroked as gently as if it were the skin of a child, and sometimes as though it were an erotic act.

"To be touched like that," said Z., a fifty-year old woman, longingly as she caressed the surface of the sand. Her movements felt erotic. She was a successful, well-to-do academic, divorced with two children, and was in an unsatisfying relationship with a married man. She was not able to leave him nor get him to devote more time to their relationship. She said that the man only left her breadcrumbs.

Z. had grown up in a large house with domestic staff but had almost always been alone. My impression was that she projected a motherly function on her lover, as is common for many women with deficient primary relationships. He did no more than the bare minimum that was necessary to maintain the relationship, and she lived in permanent, semi-conscious expectation that this would someday change. The result was constant disappointment. A clear indication of the projected primary relationship was that her daily routine, and indeed her whole life, only had meaning if she could tell *him* about it. The sun shone on her only if *he* was reachable. We had often spoken about these dynamics, and she gradually learned to pay more attention to her own needs, to be less passive and allowing towards her children, and to better accentuate her intellectual capabilities.

In her first sandplay session, Z. touched the sand lightly with her fingertips and caressed it in the sensuous manner already described. This was fascinating to watch and it created a concentrated and important silence. After a while, I noticed that the same movements had become mechanical, and her expression absent. I asked her cautiously how it felt now, and she answered that, for a moment, her thoughts had been somewhere else entirely. Where? She had just been thinking of *him* and had wondered what it would be like if he were to come see her next week. Z. had drifted into daydreams, and it had shown immediately in her movements in the sand. I tried to invite her back to the here and now, and asked her if she would like to find out what her hands wanted next. She stroked the sand again, her movements sensuous as before, but then the same thing happened again, mechanical movements and an absent expression. I asked again, and once more her thoughts had drifted away. "I imagined what it would be like to have a whole night to ourselves for once," she said. In reality, her lover didn't share this wish in the least. A few hours some afternoons were all he wanted. Such daydreams are probably similar to the fantasies of neglected children, imagining they were princesses or had rich parents. They drain life energy. Again, I tried to help Z. focus her attention on her hands' wishes, and I received a curt and sullen answer. "They don't want to caress any longer, they want to *be* caressed!"

I realised, then, what function her compulsive fantasising had. Every time the desire to be caressed arose but could not be satisfied, this dissociative state set in and Z. was no longer physically fully present. The idealising daydreams successfully prevented her from becoming aware of her real desires because it was too painful to see them go unfulfilled. Thus, one frustration was avoided, but a neurotic vicious circle had been created. The session continued. Z.'s hands lay in front of her in the sand, her face one great expression of reproach. The very tips of her fingers were buried, and it looked as if her fingers were cut off at the ends. It struck me as a physical metaphor for her life. Something was maimed because Z. could not allow herself to seize the good things in life for herself. "Your hands want to be caressed and not always do the caressing themselves," I repeated, feeling pity with those dismembered fingers. That was all I could come up with in the moment. Then I considered that she had two hands, and that one could very well caress the other. "How do your hands feel now?" I asked next. Her response came quickly, "They want to be caressed." On the one hand, Z. now had the courage to acknowledge a central yet unfulfilled need, but, on the other hand, she was stuck in a state of infantile expectancy. Like a little child that has to wait until someone will come to its aid, if indeed anyone ever does. If a child grows up in such a relationship vacuum, its reflective function will likewise be poorly developed: it is this that would allow us to speak to ourselves, for example, when we feel lonely. Z. was not able to say to her inner self, "Just nestle up and make yourself comfortable, even if *he* doesn't call you today." To initiate such an inner dialogue, a potential dialogic space must be present in the psyche, and this space is only developed if a sufficiently interacting primary-relationship figure was successfully introjected in the past. This seems not to have been the case in Z.'s life. For Z., the saviour figure, the "other," was projected outward. Only *he*, the unattainable, could free her from her loneliness, just like before, when the one irreplaceable yet inaccessible mother figure of her early childhood had not saved her from her unspeakable desolation. Her mother had suffered from severe war-related trauma all her life.

I wondered whether such a physically engrained primary care function could be made up for on a symbolic level. During the course of the sandplay session, the opposite appeared to constellate itself. The very issues that couldn't be solved repeated themselves and threatened to re-traumatise. Somewhat helpless, but relying on the "third party," on an unconscious instance, I asked, "Can the sand contribute in any way?" Suddenly, one hand slid deep into the sand and the other hand covered it on the surface. Z. seemed content. Her hands had found each other. "They're in touch with each other now," she said. "The lower hand feels the comforting weight of the upper hand distinctly, and the upper hand feels something solid below it." A first experience of physical contact. For the first time, an inner dialogue was becoming possible, from one hand to another: "I will protect you, you will protect me. You will protect me, I will protect you." Z. relaxed. The beginning of a new option of inner dialogue had not merely been expressed, it had been *experienced*. The relationship with her partner remained the same, but Z. claimed an increasing degree of autonomy in her life during the course of her therapy. She began spending a little more money on herself rather than giving *him* presents, she expanded her social life, and generally started to feel better. Her friends said she had flourished.

Beyond the Limits...

G.'s childhood was characterised by severe physical and emotional abuse until the age of four, then by his time in a children's home, until he was finally put up for international adoption at the age of nine. The first time I saw G. was three months after he had arrived in his new country.

His first activity in play was not unlike that of a two-year old. He sat on the floor in front of a shelf he could easily reach. Different types of vehicle were placed in a row on the shelf. He took one toy car after the next in his hand, regarded it from every angle, and then dropped it. G. was described to me as a child who would just run away during a walk with his adoptive parents and not come back. He would neither try to return nor did he seem to remember the way back. This left his parents understandably concerned. During the first session, G. discovered the two sandtrays and a game that he would repeat over the next few weeks: he pushed both sandtrays close to each other and let a car start driving in the one sandtray. The car then jumped and landed in the second sandtray. Little by little, G. increased the distance between the two sandtrays and the leap through the air became more dangerous for the car, the run-up longer and the outcome uncertain. From time to time, a car would plunge into the depths between the two sandtrays. I saw this as a representation of his effort, and the difficulty of which he was increasingly aware, to land in his new reality from the world of his origin. The danger, this was very clear in his depiction, was in the transition, in not being able to find solid ground beneath his feet, either here or there. I accompanied G. in therapy until he was nineteen years old and would like to describe just one session from his adolescence, when he used only dry sand for the first time. As the photo (Fig. 5) shows, he had piled up a large amount of sand to form a mountain that just reached the wooden frame of the sandtray. He had done this with infinite patience and the most delicate motor skills. The challenge had been to let more and more sand trickle on this growing mountain, but at the same time not to let any sand fall out of the sandtray, because of course this was one of the few rules during the sessions. Again and again, he looked over at me, as if to say, "You see? I can add even a little bit more. And do you see how careful I am being not to let any sand fall out of the sandtray? And successfully too, but if some should still fall out, then it was not my intention, it just happened…" And so he put all his effort into finding a balance between what was allowed and his impulse to overstep boundaries. Naturally, despite his evident best efforts, I had to spend quite some time vacuuming after the end of the session. He had enacted his new desire for transgressive behaviour and his search for limits quite literally.

I had already warned his parents at a meeting that they would likely need to prepare themselves for all sorts of behaviour from their adolescent son, but that they should not be too concerned. Not a week later, the parents found G., who hadn't come home in the evening, huddled on the ground at his bus stop after having drunk and smoked excessive amounts of alcohol and marijuana. His "friends" had left him there when he could no longer stand upright.

During further sessions of this transition period, it was interesting to observe that G. used only sand and water and would draw paths, roads and landscapes in the dry sand, as if to show me, metaphorically, what kinds of path one can travel and where they could lead. During one session, G. took very wet sand in his closed hand and let pieces of it drop back into the sandtray from quite a height. It went "*plop, plop*" and both of us immediately associated the sound with faeces dropping into the toilet. G. grinned at me mischievously and said, "It's not my fault, that's just how it sounds!!" I was put in mind of the joy and pride of a two-year old saying, "That came from me! I made that!" Regressive healing

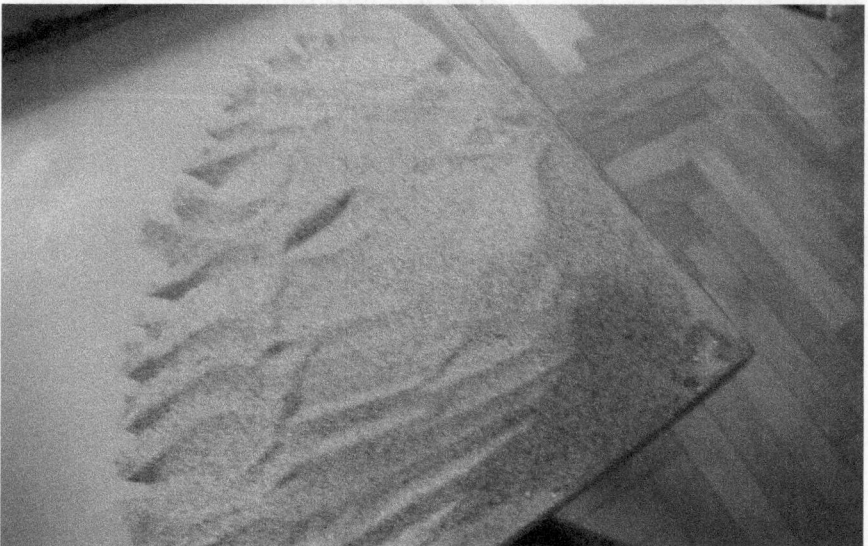

Fig. 5: Pushing boundaries

moments such as this one occur spontaneously in sandplay as part of a development process that makes up for missed opportunities in the past. This spontaneous psychic processing of severe traumas through sandplay applies to early somatic perceptions and their associated emotions. Because cognitive developmental deficits are usually also involved, additional pedagogical assistance is sometimes necessary. In G.'s case, the Feuerstein method proved beneficial.

Eros

From the very first moment, touching the sand's surface had an erotic quality for F., a musician in his forties. "I enjoy compressing the sand; I can really feel how things come together and result in a form. Stroking across it is like touching the skin of a woman, in different places even. I like that I can create something like the body of a woman, her breasts, for example, or her belly." Here, F. was in control of the situation and could enjoy his active role. With his partner, on the other hand, the exact opposite happened. Though they had a good relationship on the whole, the active role expected of him in their sexuality triggered an inhibiting pressure to perform. Savouring the eroticism in the sand, meanwhile, had a calming and energising effect on F. He said, "It is so nice to make these motions and gestures without any aim or purpose whatsoever, just for the pure joy in the movements themselves!"

What are the Variables?

A scientist in his sixties with a brilliant career, who didn't have the slightest problem taking weekly intercontinental flights to lecture at conferences, found himself entangled in inconsistencies between his successful professional life and his failing relationships with women. W. said of himself, "I think I just lack sensibility in interpersonal relationships. I'm not a sensitive person, I'm a bit like a bulldozer." Since I could scarcely get a word in edgewise during the sessions, I asked him if it was possible that he occasionally got bored when other people were speaking. The answer came faster than expected: "Yes, exactly! I am bored to death!" Although listening clearly wasn't his strength, he did possess a thirst for knowledge and a pioneering spirit. I suggested using the sandtray as an exercise to discover his own sensibility. I invited him to do no more than lay his hands on the sand at first and to listen and concentrate on how this contact felt. W. didn't need to be told twice. In next to no time, he was sitting at the sandtray with his eyes closed. I didn't interrupt, although I wasn't certain he had actually listened to my instructions. After a while, he said the sand felt cold. I invited him to linger at this perception and to try to listen if there was anything particular his hands wanted. W. didn't move his hands one bit, his face and posture showing an utmost of concentration. After a while, he opened his eyes and I asked him how it had felt. He answered, "First the sand was cold, then it changed. It felt like a human body, as if there had been skin and a living body underneath." W. appeared moved and, above all, puzzled by this brief event that had just taken place inside him. "So," he continued, "what were the variables?" He was asking himself what the critical factors had been to get from the perception of "cold" to the perception of "living body." In the end, we agreed there had been at least three variables: listening, being silent, and not wanting anything in particular.

Closeness and Distance

With the following three sequences, I would like to show how working with the sand can also be integrated in non-analytical sessions under certain circumstances. A trainee psychotherapist was keen to try a brief self-experience in sandplay because she wanted to get to know this medium. I suggested selecting an issue from her current life situation, to which we would devote four sessions. Thus, we had set a specific focus from the outset. The sessions were to consist of one part conversation and one part sandplay. I had provided a few select miniatures, but as we will see, R. used only dry sand. She wanted to use the sessions to work on a situation with her partner, which was causing her headaches at the time. On the one hand she wanted to move in with him, but on the other hand she was concerned for her freedom, of loosing her independence, and running the risk of adjusting too much to his habits. We spoke about these concerns, and for the last third of each session she also worked in the sand. R. moved her hands in a similar manner in all three sessions, but with a different result each time. The traces of these movements in the sand shed light on the non-verbal, somatic dialogue that R. entered into with herself and that helped her to a new degree of clarity regarding her dilemma. Working with the sand can be likened to a sensorial, kinesthetic narrative, which has its own momentum and helps to bring the conscious and unconscious together, thereby having a regulating effect on the psyche.

Figure 6 shows the traces of both hands running from top to bottom. As R. commented unprompted, they come very close to each other but most definitely should not touch. While working in

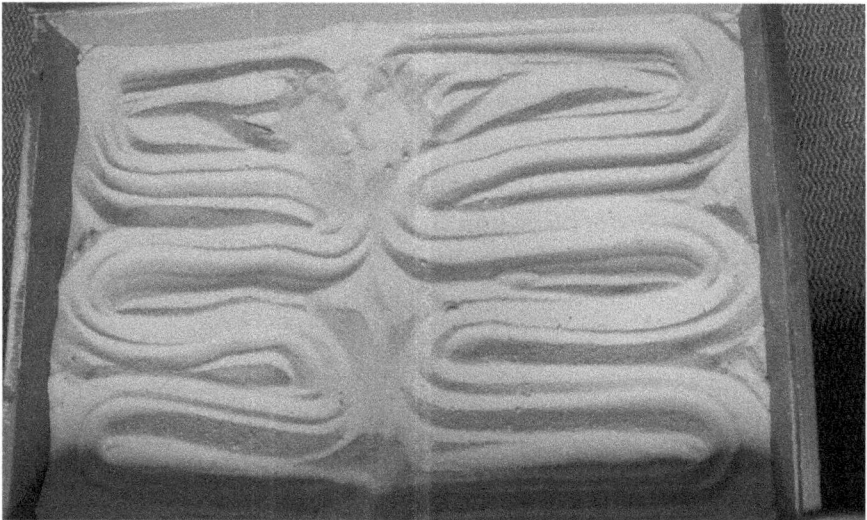

Fig. 6: Closeness and distance - Session 1

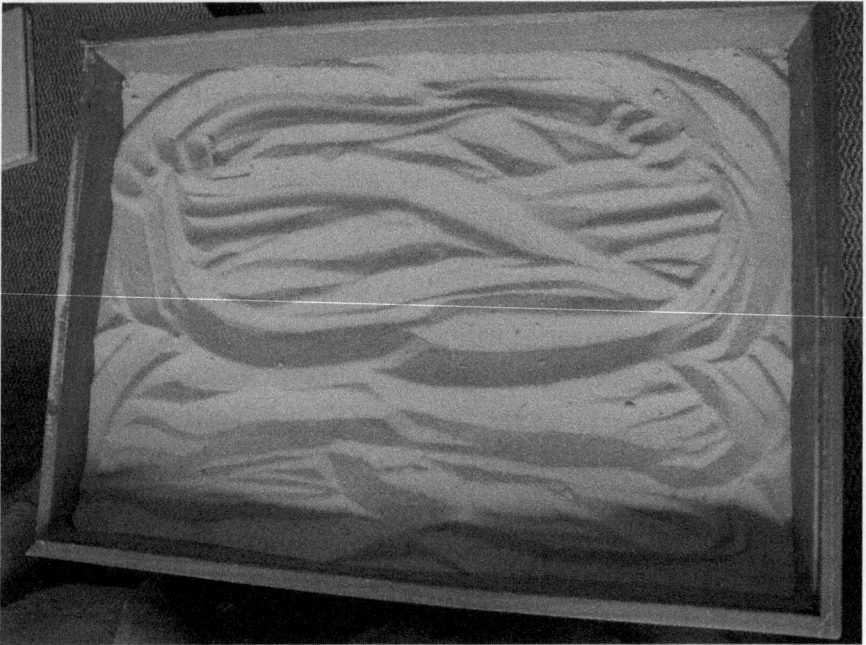

Fig. 7: Closeness and distance - Session 2

the sand she had kept a very close eye on these approaches, and she was glad that they had turned out just as she wanted. We can see that both hands only used their respective half of the available space. Each remained in its own territory, as it were; the right hand on the right and the left hand on the left. R. was relieved at the end of the session. As mentioned above, we made no connection between her drawing in the sand and the topic of closeness and distance in a relationship, about which we had spoken extensively just previously. Had we done so, her following sandwork would likely have been influenced, and who knows if it would have unfolded with the same spontaneity. For example, after the second session R. was not aware that her movements had been entirely different than in the first. It is plain to see in Figure 7: her hands crossed one another, each exploring the entire available space in its own manner. The lines come together, everything is entwined, joined, and intermingled.

In the third session, the kinesthetic narrative reaches a further stage: the lines again flow across the entire area, but in parallel this time. R.'s movements had been just the same, her hands moving freely in all directions but neither crossing, nor merging, nor avoiding contact with each other. It made an impression of two forces cooperating, and the image conveys a sense of harmony. Whether these combined energies are a metaphor for a functioning relationship, or whether the images portrayed R.'s own contrasting psychic energies coming together here in the final image, is not relevant – one does not exclude the other. Here, again, we can assume that matter and psyche will work together, that soul and body speak a common language: as within, so without, as above, so below.

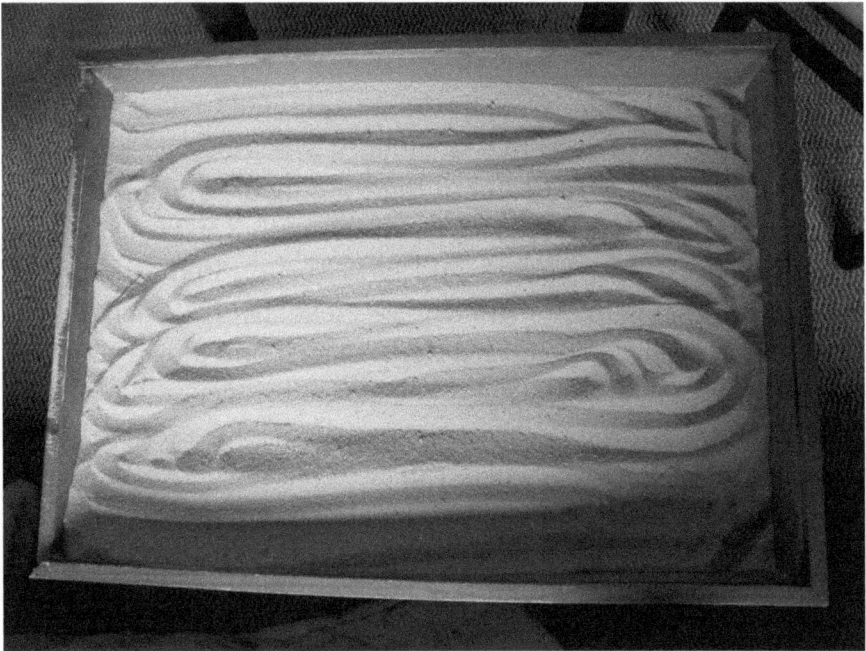

Fig. 8: Closeness and distance - Session 3

Transformation

Sometimes patients try to understand individual elements in their image on a cognitive level, either during its creation or as soon as it is finished, and expect the therapist to help interpret possible meanings. This bears the risk of symbolic meanings being missed, if they cannot yet be grasped in the moment and would require more time and maybe a more associative view to establish themselves in conscious form. One would settle for a metaphoric level, which might well have its own effectiveness but doesn't even come close to the revolutionary effect inherent in a living symbol. Thus, the therapist sometimes has to protect the patient from an overhasty desire to classify the created image into known categories, or else the transformative potential of a symbol, which always comprises strong emotions from both sides, might not unfold its full effect.

With the following short example of two sandplay sessions in a group session I would like to show the profound existential effect sandplay can have aside from its therapeutic effect. I developed the group setting for prospective facilitators of expressive sandwork; it has also proven very useful in the training of aspiring psycho-therapists and can be offered to all interested persons after a degree of preparatory work and with certain limitations. The group setting involves eight to, at most, twelve participants working on two consecutive days in dyads: one player and one empathic, silent witness. One of these sessions generally lasts an hour, after which the roles are switched, silent witnesses becoming players. Finally, the experiences can be discussed within the group in a verbal follow-up – but only as extensively and in as much detail as each player wishes – or not at all, if individual participants prefer. If there is an uneven number of participants, one of the group's instructors can take part so that each participant has a partner. This was the case in the session that I would like to describe here. U., the participant with whom I formed a dyad, was a vivacious, inquisitive woman of advanced years, who had clearly already done some therapeutic work on herself and was willing to face this potentially very personal experience. Her strong emotional involvement was apparent in her expression from the beginning, and I mirrored it in my own physical and emotional state. From the selection of available miniatures, U. had chosen some houses, fences and trees. I could see that it was important to her to erect protective fences and demarcations. She kept changing them, because they were either too constricting or too permeable. There was something heavy and sinister in the air but without concrete expression. Towards the end of the session – after much deliberation, trial, and hesitation – U. finally placed a menacing figure in the sand in one corner, and the whole scene was given a narrative context. My intense countertransference reactions – shifting between joy, fear, disgust, tension, and anger – relaxed some-what after this gesture, and gave way to a sense of achievement. U.'s verbal explanation followed before the session was finished. She had tried to summarise her life story in broad outline: it had started with a childhood trauma, which influenced her life for decades but which she had been able to process with tremendous effort. Today, she was grateful for her life and was content.

The second session took place the following day. This time U. hadn't fetched any miniatures. She sat motionless in front of the sandtray for a long time, and it was clear that she had no idea what she wanted to do with it. She sat there, expectant, her hands leaving a few traces in the dry sand. It was as if she was saying, "I already told the story of my life last time, and it was good; but what should I do now?" U. started drawing a rectangle in the sand and removing a little sand from within it. At first I felt a certain sense of expectation and curiosity, but then it was joined by unease and fear, and suddenly I had a clear and frightening thought: she is digging her own grave. U. redid the edges of the narrow rectangle again and again, carefully and patiently, because the dry sand kept trickling in from the top. Unlike the previous day, where an inner conflict had been apparent, her gestures now expressed determination and also a meditative calm, while my own psychophysical system was quivering with excitement and fear. "To build her own grave? What courage!", I thought, and scarcely dared breathe. At the same time, I considered that this idea may just have sprung from my own imagination and that U. might actually be making something entirely different, maybe the foundations of a house. But these alternative ideas did not last long, and it became ever clearer that it was a grave and not just somebody's grave but her own. Now I feared the moment that she would put something (but what?) inside it. But nothing happened. The rectangle was just there; and not even in the centre of the sandtray but offset to the left and lower side, which only increased the image's expressiveness. Minutes passed, half an hour had passed and U. did nothing but sit in silent contemplation of this image. Then she stood up, walked over to the table with the miniatures and fetched some small, white doves. These doves are from my personal collection of miniatures and they are particularly dear to me. I brought a large number of them back from Colombia, where I had worked with children whose families had been victims of the armed conflict. I then took these doves with me to Palestine, Ukraine, Kuala Lumpur,

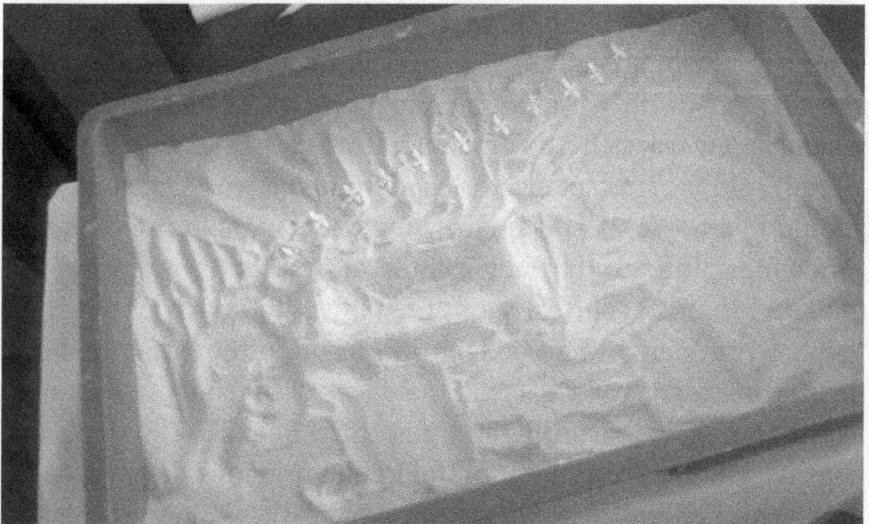

Fig. 9: The empty grave

and Germany, where they are today used in countless sandplay images. While my thoughts were wandering off, U. had placed eleven of these doves in a diagonal emanating from the top edge of the rectangle. It looked as if the birds were leaving the hole in the ground in soaring flight. Of the sandtray's rather modest three dimensions, this effect had expanded the third, the endless sky opening up overhead. After regarding this image for another long time, U. looked up at me and asked, "Do you know what that is?" I nodded. She continued, "But the grave is empty, the doves have flown away," and she added the quote from the Gospel of John 8:32, "And you shall know the truth, and the truth shall make you free".

A few months later, when we came to speak about that image again, U. told me that she had also perceived the hole as a bathtub and that it had reminded her of C. G. Jung's description of the alchemical treatise Rosarium Philosophorum. It had been important to her to add a lot of doves to the image because they expressed skyward movement.

A Therapeutic Gesture

In a psychiatric children's hospital in Shanghai, sandplay was used to treat children with autistic symptoms, both in individual sessions and in groups. During a supervision session, one of the therapists and I came to speak about the case of a child with aggressive behaviour. The therapist asked me what she should do if a child continuously and purposefully threw sand out of the sandtray. I had no general answer for such a case and asked her, if only to better understand the situation, how she herself had reacted to this behaviour. The experienced and kindhearted therapist showed me her hands opened in a holding gesture: "I tried to catch the sand like this, and to throw it back in the sandtray." When the child noticed this, it stopped for a while. But

71

the most important thing was that the child also looked the therapist in the eyes for the very first time. The child had received a momentarily adequate response to its offered behaviour. Its overflowing emotion, just like the overflowing sand, had been caught in the friendliest of manners. The therapist's gesture must have surprised the child and thus paved the way to perceiving reality one step further.

Coldness

"Oh, how cold the sand feels! I hadn't expected that. I thought the sand would be warm because it is warm in this room. But the sand is cold and hard." Almost startled by this discovery, O. lifted the palms of her hands from the sand and instead drew some lines with the tips of her index fingers. It was a hot summer day and the sand was completely dry; it could not objectively be cold. The startling sense of coldness must have had a very deep connection to events in O.'s biography. I did not comment on this. The lines she had started to draw began to take shape: there were two symmetrical oval forms with beautiful decorations inside them. She called it a butterfly, but, as she pointed out to me, upon closer inspection the butterfly had one broken wing and the small decorations actually appeared more like little holes in the wings. This first session ended with a feeling of disappointment. She had hoped that sandplay would reveal something positive, when, in fact, it had pointed more to her problems than to her resources.

O. appeared to be a strong and sensitive person who had accomplished a lot in her life. She was successful in her profession and had a grown-up son from a former marriage. In spite of this, her first contact with the sand had revealed a fragile and precarious side which would need to be worked on. Much later during the course of her therapy, the sense of "cold" turned out to be a recurring theme in her life. The day of her birth had been the coldest in 50 years, and, as a newborn, she had diarrhea for two weeks. But instead of being cared for by her mother, she was taken care of by her emotionally very distant and strict grandmother. Family members said of her as a small child that she would remain seated motionless in one place if told to do so, without daring to move until the grandmother allowed it. She also recounted a recent dream about her boyfriend that had revolved around the theme of temperature.

In her dream, as in reality, she had an electric heater, and this heater was broken. In her dream, she asked her boyfriend if he could fix it. He agreed and promptly removed the heating element, which was indeed the broken part in her dream, and said, "There, now it's fixed." O. wondered in her dream how this could be because the heating element was precisely what the heater required to produce warmth. She woke up.

At first, we had commented this dream on an objective level, describing the relationship unsparingly but also humorously. The boyfriend was keeping his emotional distance and kept conveying to her that her desire for closeness and intimacy was excessive, which naturally unsettled her. Thus, adjusting to him meant renouncing her own emotions. The fact that she had already experienced such a situation in her early childhood, in her relationship with her emotionally icy grandmother, only emerged gradually. Another striking element in this dream was that *she* had asked her partner to repair the heater. We could interpret this as an unconscious expectation that the relationship repair her own lacking capacity for warmth and empathy towards herself (the heater in need of repair). Her relationship with this man ended gradually over the following years. This lengthy phase of separation revealed how strongly she had projected a profound, archetypical need for care, protection, and her right to existence on her partner. As long as the relationship had held, no matter how unsatisfied both partners were, neither O. nor I, as the therapist, could fully grasp the intensity of the neglect she had experienced in her early childhood. The relationship shielded her from feeling

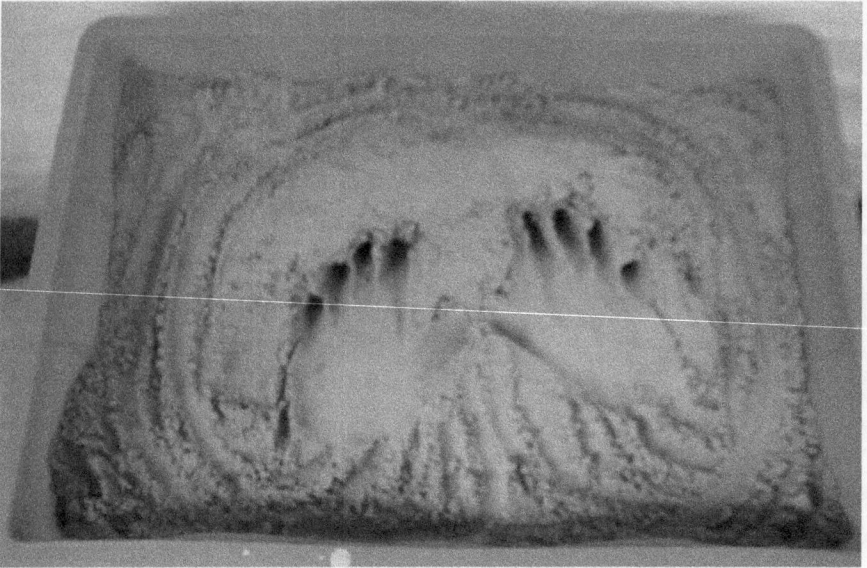

Fig. 10: Holding tight

both the existential helplessness and fear for her life that she must have repeatedly had as a child.

Holding tight and being held

After a year in which sandplay had become an integral part of her analytic therapy, there came a number of very intense sessions revealing the full extent of the "coldness" problem. O. had made great progress towards psychic autonomy and felt a lot better. Unlike in her previous sessions, she now frequently chose the wet sand and made a point of digging deep into it to feel its firmness. In one session, she said that it did her good to hold on to something. She reached deep into the sand and compressed it in her fists. She said that holding something tight like that also felt like being held. She was holding, but she also felt held herself. She repeated this behaviour over a number of sessions. Once again, O. dug both hands into the damp sand, holding it tight, and remained motionless for a while. But this time her expression changed. She looked worried, then distressed, and frightened. I asked her how she was feeling, but she didn't answer. Then I saw tears running down her cheeks, dripping into the cold, wet sand, while her hands were still buried motionlessly in the sand. The palpable sensation of coldness, obstruction, and forlornness could not have been more dramatic. Everything was freezing, wet, and hopeless. What I was witnessing here was an early-childhood experience of catastrophic abandonment. For a brief moment, I myself felt an impulse to leave the room and to leave O. alone. The archaic child's fear of tumbling into nothingness had been constellated in myself as well. The self-regulation of the psyche was gridlocked. O.'s tears kept falling into the sand; it seemed to me as if they would never stop. Her body looked as though it were being tortured. I touched her on the shoulder and handed her a paper tissue. It felt far too thin and pitifully inadequate to make any difference to her state. As if in slow motion, O. drew one hand out of the sand and began to blow her nose. This released her from the blockage. After she had recovered somewhat, we spoke for a long time about what had happened. She described how she had suddenly had the clear sensation that, though she herself could hold tight to the sand, she would immediately fall into an abyss the moment her hands let go. She could no longer move and was incapable even of thinking. She had never experienced anything of the sort.

Sandplay was out of the question for the next few months because the sandtray with wet sand frightened her. Various episodes of abandonment and fear of death from different stages in her life came up during the next few sessions.

It took a while for O.'s interest in sandplay to return, and she decided to work in the dry sand first. She soon felt the familiar impulse to hold tight, but this time she could do it in a playful form: she had realised that she needn't hold on to the sand with all her might, rather she could control how tightly she clenched her hands. Something had clearly changed in her psychophysical state, and her infantile fear of not being held did not materialise. She could now hold the sand tight and also let it go again. She had thereby discovered her own capacity for control over her environment, and also regained a great deal of self-efficacy. She pushed the sand together to form a flat mound and smoothed its surface. It was a hard, solid structure. She repeated a similar sequence in the next session. Again, the round, compact mound arose out of the sand, its surface particularly soft from the mixture of sand and water. It felt like silk, and O. was clearly moved and content to let her hands stroke across it repeatedly. Then she made two brushing movements from the centre of the mound, one to the upper left and one to the upper right. She regarded the result for a long time and then exclaimed, "Oh, a child's face with raised hands!" Indeed, the image now resembled just that. The mound was the round head of a small child raising its little arms trustingly towards the observer. "I would like to have been like that," O. added, "cheerful and embracing the world with open arms." One could say that this symbolic experience had activated both O.'s motherly function

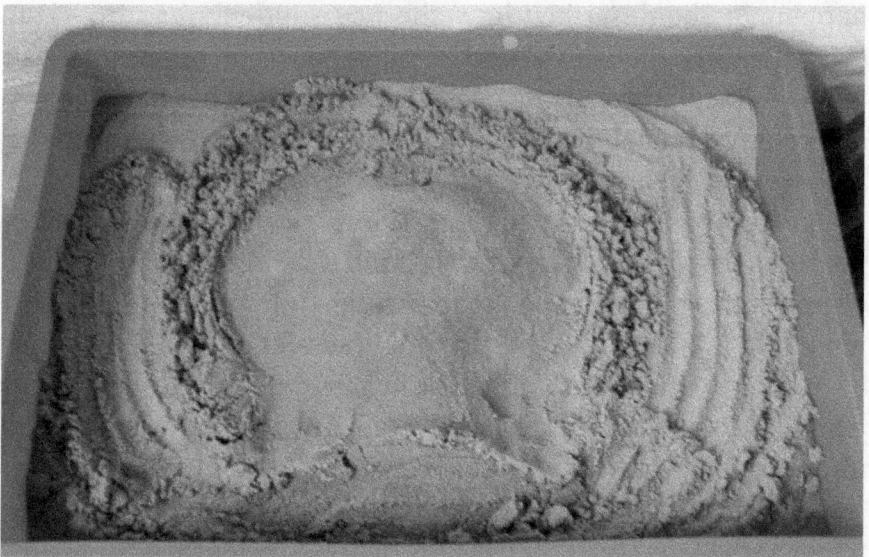

Fig. 11: A little girl

(positive mother archetype) and her own vitality, spontaneity, and creativity (child archetype).

Her sand creations continued. O. generally became more playful during the sessions. There were further variations on the theme of the compact mound. This time it was high and broad, and she had started pounding on it with the palms of her hands. She beat it rhythmically, and it sounded like a drum. She smiled to herself and kept drumming – louder, slower, faster. It was fascinating to listen to, and I was so taken with the different tones and her harmonious movements that it was almost like being torn from a trance when she suddenly stopped and opened her eyes. "Already finished?", I asked. "Yes." "And how did it feel?" "Wonderful, just wonderful. I could have kept drumming like that for hours." "And what made you stop? We still have a lot of time." "I thought to myself: here I am in therapy, and we should probably be speaking to each other. It might be a waste of time to just keep drumming away." I proposed that she trust in her expressed feeling that she could "keep drumming like that for hours." So she closed her eyes again and found her rhythm once more. Then I saw that her right hand was moving more slowly and gradually, as if in slow motion, and then remained lying on the sand. I watched her left hand slowly rise and fall a few more times, as if it were a ceremonious act. O. must have been deeply moved by something. When she opened her eyes after a long silence, she told me what had happened.

At first she had enjoyed the rhythm, as had I. Then she had begun to feel as if the mound in the sand were her own body, her shoulder, to be exact. Then she had felt a hand, her own, on her right shoulder and on the sand mound at the same time, and it had felt good. And she had understood that it was actually the hand of her father, the same father who had criticised her all of his life and who was never satisfied with anything she did. Now his hand was resting on her shoulder in her mind, and this gesture told her, "It's all right. You are good just the way you are. You don't have to be any different. You are perfect as you are." It was like a fatherly blessing. She had felt everything in her body relax and let go. Finally, she was allowed to be how she wanted. In the following weeks, she often remembered how her father's hand had felt on her shoulder, and it felt as if this approving, fatherly blessing were accompanying her through her daily life.

The fact that the shoulder had simultaneously been a form in the sand, and the hand of her father simultaneously her own, and that she had performed a ceremony on herself that she had not experienced in her childhood and adolescence, all this illustrates the complex, subtle, and creative ways the self-regulation of the psyche can take the lead. My verbal interventions were kept to a minimum, only the occasional "And how is that now?" and "How does that feel?" I made no attempts to interpret or explain the occurrences in the sand. At most I attempted mirroring or paraphrasing, as if to ask "have I understood that correctly?" when the patient shared an element of her feelings. In an extreme emergency, when O. wasn't able to extricate herself from her paralysis, a gesture had proved helpful. As did the question whether she wouldn't like to continue, when she had interrupted her playful and exploring actions too soon.

The importance of a stable transference relationship during such processes is self-evident. Equally, it goes without saying that the therapist may not always be prepared to go along with such intense processes, and that the wish to use sandplay during a session must come from both sides.

The Owl's Gaze

Here I would like to follow up with a sequence of images that show the effect of the self-regulation of the psyche in the case of severe traumas. Z.'s childhood was marked by extreme poverty. From the age of 6, her parents sent her to sell flowers in restaurants. Despite her deprivations, she had been able to study later in life because her teachers had advocated for her. She had become a successful psychotherapist and was happy with her profession, but she suffered from a row of psychosomatic symptoms.

The sandplay sessions I would like to describe here were preceded by verbal sessions to establish a case history and to build trust in the therapeutic relationship.

Z. wished to learn sandplay for her own practice and was prepared to engage in a process of her own. In her first sandplay session, she formed a landscape with a lake in the middle, surrounded by trees and green spaces. Sitting at the shore of the lake were a man and a woman. Z. said this was a place where one could relax. In the upper right corner of the sandtray, Z. had carefully placed the sun, moon, and stars made of gold paper. Z. was happy with her work; she particularly liked these celestial bodies. They reminded me of a Brothers Grimm tale in which an orphan child is travelling alone and asks the sun, moon, and stars for help. The sun scorches the child, the moon wants to eat her, and only the stars take pity on her. I kept this association to myself. The

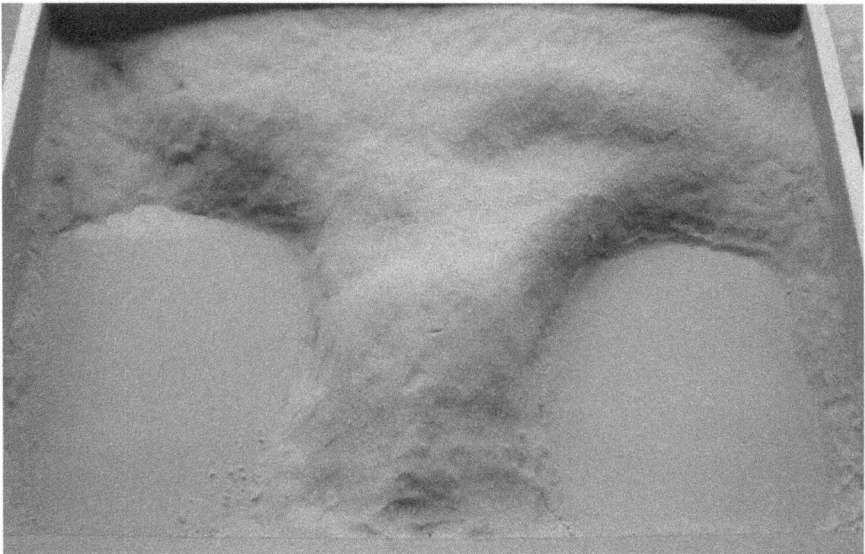

Fig. 12: An eery face 1

entire scene felt pleasant, the vegetation was fresh, and yet there was also a certain sense of distance. I had the impression that Z. still needed to build more trust before she would be able to engage in anything more difficult.

In the following session, Z. began using only the sand. She churned up the whole area a couple of times and then created an image that on the one hand could have shown two lakes separated by a ridge, or on the other hand a broad, eery nose section between two large, unseeing eyes. (Fig. 12)

I didn't comment on the image. She herself said that she didn't know what it was. The image gave me an uneasy feeling either way. It appeared empty and stifling at the same time. But I had no idea, explanation, or hypothesis, and no particular motivation to search for one. Z. made very similar images in the next two sessions. Both times the image could be seen as a landscape with two lakes, or, and this was becoming ever clearer, as a face with a very frightening, almost monstrous gaze. The second of these images,

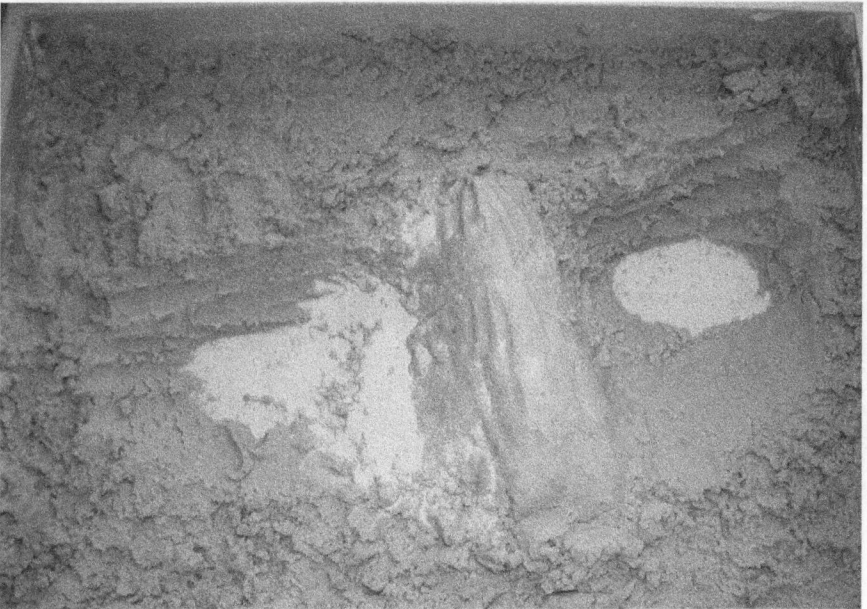

Fig. 13: An eery face 2

where Z. had used wet sand, made a particularly heavy and inaccessible impression. She had been concentrated in her work and the atmosphere had been tense, an impression that I would never have verbalised since it emanated from the image itself. The next session was approaching, scheduled as usual for the evening. Already by early afternoon I was feeling tired. The closer Z.'s session came, the clearer I felt an inner aversion to my profession. I would have liked nothing more than to go home at once and cancel Z.'s appointment. A part of me hoped she wouldn't come, and I fantasised how she might forget the appointment. In that moment, I made no connection between my feelings and the content of her sandplay. When Z. rang the doorbell on time and entered the counselling room I noticed her withdrawn expression. Or was it just my prejudiced imagination? A tense air filled the room. Then Z. told me, and it was clear how difficult this was for her, that she would like to work in the sand again, but with her back turned to me. She placed the sandtray so that she faced away from me when she sat in front of it. Instead, she now had the shelves of countless miniature figures in front of her. She sat motionless at the sandtray for a long time and didn't reach for a single one of the figures.

Then Z. began drawing circles with both hands, but she appeared to be exerting such pressure that it made a loud, unpleasant grinding noise. She drew the circles in sweeping movements away from herself, the rhythm already hectic and becoming ever faster, more hasty and restless. I wished she would stop, but she kept circling further and faster, the noise turning to a screech. I could hear Z.'s breathing. She was exerting herself physically, there was clearly a sense of rage and hate, and she just wouldn't stop. I guessed, as I could still only see her back, that she was wearing herself out, sweating and completely out of breath. After what seemed like an unbearably long time, Z.'s movements finally came to a halt. She cried. Her shoulders heaved and she sobbed. I waited because I felt that she still needed physical

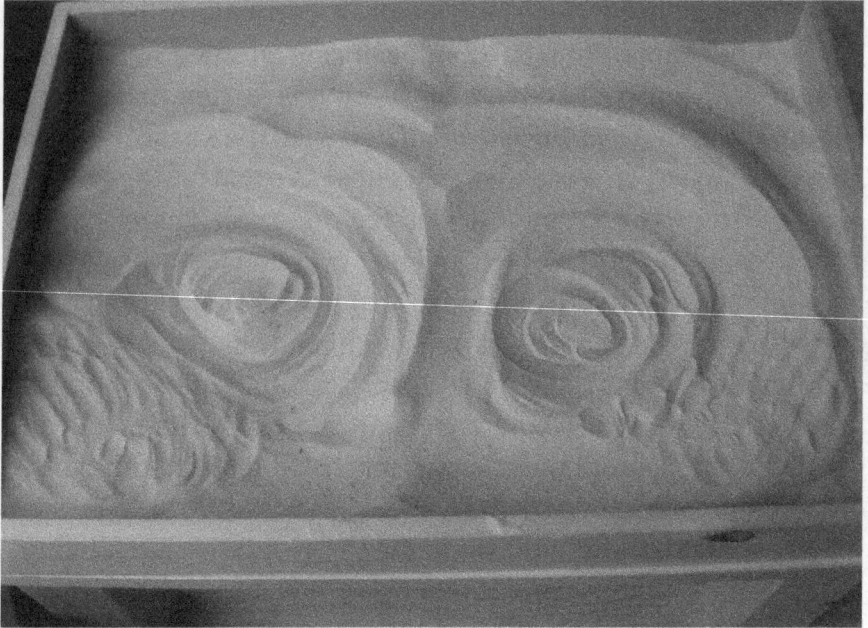

Fig. 14: Working through the trauma

distance and would have perceived any approach on my part as an intrusion. Then Z. stood up and took a seat in the therapy chair, where we normally spoke. She was still crying. Slowly, she began to tell me how she had nearly become a victim of rape as a child, something she had never told anyone before, not even her husband. I asked her if she hadn't felt too alone in front of the sandtray, since she had decided to turn her back to me. She answered that being alone had felt necessary because of her immense sense of shame. But she had still felt in good company and well cared for, not by me as the therapist, because I had to remain in the distant background, but by the miniature figures and objects in front of her on the shelves. They had been a comforting presence and just what she needed. She had felt protected by them.

Such a cathartic, motoric and sensorial re-experience of the trauma through the medium of sand would never have been possible with words alone. The trauma first had to be reactivated physically in all of its horror before it could be narrated. The sand is the tool that helps the body to actively set this re-experience in scene. Z.'s sessions progressed, we continued to speak about the issue, and she processed it further with the help of the sandtray. In the following months, there were two sessions in which Z. resumed her dual circles. In the first of these sessions, Z. drew a lying eight or the mathematical symbol for infinity in the dry sand with her index finger. Following the course of this symbol with her finger created an almost hypnotic atmosphere that Z. said she found dizzying and calming. I perceived this movement as part of a process aiming to outgrow the trauma, to lift it above the level of individual fate and extreme personal injustice. Some weeks later, there was a profound transformation of the problem which found its symbolic and kinesthetic expression in Z.'s sandwork. She began moving her hands in circles again, but this time the movement was focused and controlled. The circles changed directions. The whole thing had a playful feeling this time, but still retained a certain focus and determination. The two well-drawn circles, which had now appeared in the semi-dry sand, had nothing random or unintended about them. They seemed like a determined expression of Z.'s self-efficacy, conveying clarity and strength. Finally, Z. looked for two small, dark blue glass beads and placed one in the centre of each of the circles. Then she added a little triangular indentation between the two circles and all of a sudden there were two large owl's eyes gazing at us intently from the sandtray. The gaze was dark as the night where the owls rule. The little beak appeared precise and sharp, clearly indicating a bird of prey. Z. was so taken with this image that she wanted to photograph it and carry it with her in her handbag in the future. (Fig. 15) We spoke about the fact that the owl was dedicated to the goddess Athena in ancient Greece and is still considered a symbol of female wisdom until today. We discovered that Z. had recently achieved a new capacity for differentiation of all things dark. It allowed her to recognise the dark sides of those around her early on and to

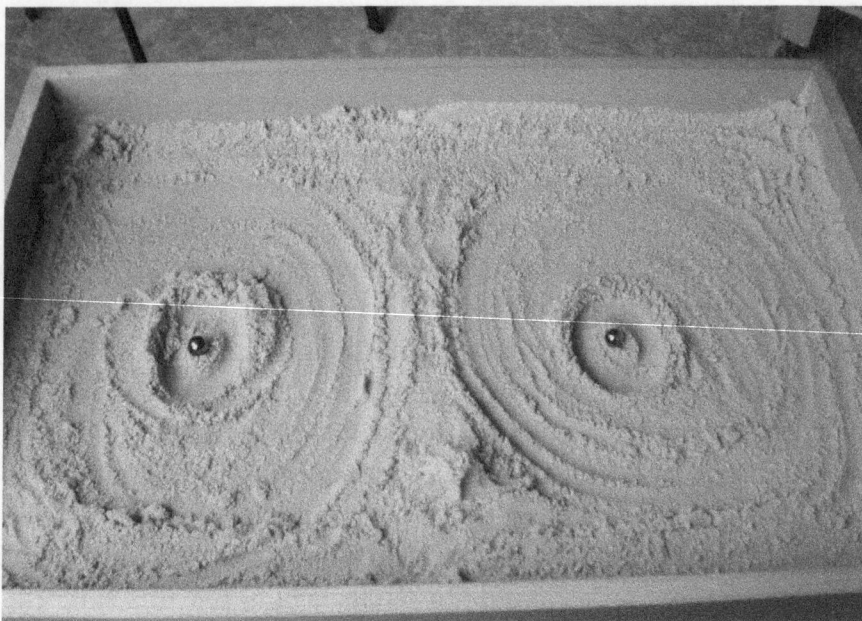

Fig. 15: The owl's gaze

either avoid concrete dangers in life, or to better confront them. The nocturnal bird of prey arose out of our words and associations in all its strength and majestic beauty. Over the following months, Z. observed profound changes in her state of mind and in her work as a therapist. She had become more self-confident, was scarcely afraid of authoritative behaviour, no longer cared what others thought of her, was less impulsive and quick-tempered, and had become more patient with her male patients, with a greater willingness to listen to them. This process had clearly effected a considerable shift in her psyche. Z. now used her raptor's gaze to protect herself in her native cultural context in which gender roles were extremely polarised. Her social and political engagement made her a catalyst for young women in her home country, who otherwise ran the risk of becoming permanently stuck in a victim role. From then on, she carried the owl's gaze as an actual talisman, inside and outside, wherever she went.

THIRD CHAPTER

Self-regulation of the Psyche
in Individual Sandplay Therapy

Over the following pages, I would like to use a therapy situation in an individual setting to describe how a child's psyche is able to regulate itself even after multiple severe traumas, provided a free and protected space for symbolic expression is available. It will become clear how little verbal intervention on behalf of the therapist can be necessary and how much communication occurs from body to body.

The therapeutic method in the sandplay sessions of this ten-year-old adopted boy was very similar to the method of expressive sandwork, which is described in the following chapters. Expressive sandwork is a specific method of psychosocial intervention which can be practised by lay volunteers in a group setting. This necessarily implicates that the adult facilitators accompanying each child's sandplay must do without therapeutic intervention and cannot ask questions or otherwise encourage verbal exchange. In this specific situation that I would like to describe here, an individual setting as we have established, verbal communication was precluded for other reasons. From the beginning, the boy barely reacted when addressed. He appeared blocked as soon as I even looked at him. Thus, not being spoken to was his precondition for beginning therapy. Once I had accepted this, his process of pictorial, symbolic expression made remarkable progress. What is more, I was able to gain valuable insight into the psyche's functioning: as if through a microscope, I observed the child's psyche gradually begin to extricate itself from a gridlocked situation caused by multiple underlying traumas, and to make up for deficiently experienced developmental phases in early childhood through symbolic play and through the experience of relationship with the therapist.

First, I will summarise a few fundamental principles of sandplay therapy according to Dora Kalff (1960). According to Kalff, if the therapist notices that certain content in a child's play could be connected to current or past experiences in its life, they do not verbalise this. Such an intervention would interfere with the unconsciously governed course of play and might confront the child too soon or too painfully with something that is not yet ready to be confronted. Furthermore, an intervention aimed at a meta level would overlook the significance and value of the symbolic play as it is, by viewing symbolic play as a metaphor for something else, something underlying. For a child, however, play in itself is both thinking and problem solving. For a playing child, symbolic play incorporates everything that is needed. It is deeply rooted existentially, neurobiologically embedded in the subcortical structures (Panksepp, 1998), and has its own timing. Just like organic growth, symbolic play cannot be rushed. In sandplay, the therapist observes the child's play processes and tries to read their symbolic levels. But rather than relating merely cognitively to content, the therapist also acts as a resonance body for the associated emotional level. We assume that the child perceives this integrated relatedness implicitly and on an unconscious level, and that new insights and experiences are thereby opened up from the inside. A child instinctively tries new relationship models in play (in the sense of the operative models described by Bowlby (1969)), which it will then also apply in the outside world and which can thereby become anchored in its personality. As long as all this can take effect in sandplay, there is almost no need for verbal exchange. If, however, the child has lost interest in sandplay and/or its play content has repeated itself unvaried for a lengthy period of time, then the therapist will need to resort to additional therapeutic methods. If and when sandplay reaches its limitations depends on the age of the child and on the type and degree of the mental health problem. One of the great advantages of sandplay is that the child builds trust in the therapeutic situation early on and also quickly experiences a great degree of self-efficacy. The therapist recognise the child as the expert of its own play. This initiates a spontaneous, resource-oriented process. Once inner resources have manifested themselves and are available to the child as new energetic potential and as a newly acquired capacity to judge situations, then development can be made up for. Children with neurotic disorders have good chances of recovery with sandplay. The precondition is that advisory talks are also held with the parents in parallel. For childhood dissociative disorders, sandplay according to Kalff (1960) is not sufficient in itself. It can, however, be integrated into a more complex therapy process. In the case of adolescents and young adults, it is often necessary to integrate sandplay into a preceding and subsequent verbal part of therapy sessions. Nevertheless, even in these situations, the symbolic content of a completed sand image is not discussed in the same session. Again, we assume that the symbols carry an excess of meaning, which must be given time to act further, and which cannot immediately be translated into a more conscious form. The therapist will, however, mirror and also discuss emotions, thoughts, and perceptions described by the patient during or after sandplay. Every sand image acts on a number of levels, on the somatic, emotional, psychic, and spiritual. Each of these levels could, in theory, be interpreted and amplified during each play process. The therapist's task here is to understand what the patient needs most in the moment, and which level is relevant. The role of silent witness is always the first and most important. All further interpretative courses of action emanate from that role, adjusted to the needs of the patient.

The ten-year-old boy, who was adopted when he was 22 months old, was accompanied to my practice by his father because of the boy's non-compliant and obstinate behaviour. One talk with both parents about the boy's case history had preceded this encounter. When I saw U. for the first time, I could feel the responsibility building inside me. I was overcome with anxiety as to my therapeutic skills, as I had never experienced before. I wondered if this feeling of inadequacy inside me was proportional to the unfulfilled needs of the boy and if it also mirrored something that his parents likely felt in their interactions with him and that he himself, most of all, would have felt. "Insufficient" – this must have been the baseline situation of his early childhood. The sentence "I can't do it, it's not possible" seemed to be one that U. not only carried around with him but also provoked in other people as a kind of countertransference reaction.

U.'s anamnesis showed that he had been transferred to a children's hospital by the family doctor at the age of three months, due to underweight and a broken rib and leg. The x-ray revealed further partially healed fractures of the arm and nasal bone. Suspicions of extreme physical abuse were confirmed. Mother and son were relocated to sheltered accommodation. Hopes that the mother would establish a satisfactory relationship with her child were not fulfilled during the following eight months. Nothing is known of the mother's diagnosis. At the age of eight months, U. was taken in by a foster family, where he received adequate and warm-hearted care. Only a year later, at the age of 22 months and once he must have already established a stable bond with his foster mother, he was offered up for adoption. Finding himself in a new family was a great shock for U., and he would cry in his new adoptive parents' house for weeks on end. He would also vomit frequently, especially at night. He suffered chronic constipation and was prone to infections. Crying often merged into vomiting and vice versa. The parents felt helpless a lot of the time, and the child seemed inconsolable. Photos from this time show U. with a dulled expression, his adoptive parents next to him, valiantly doing the best they could, but the depressive prevailing mood of disappointment and pain cannot be overlooked. Only gradually did U. adjust to the new situation. He first became attuned to the father, who offered him a lot of physical closeness, then gradually also to the mother, an empathic, hardworking woman who worked as a primary school teacher. To everyone's great surprise, U.'s adoptive mother became pregnant one and a half years later. There followed a total of three siblings in brief intervals over the next few years, two boys and a girl. Today, U. is a gaunt looking boy with large, melancholy eyes and an anxious expression. The skinny hands, the hanging head, the adults' questions he left unanswered, all this reminded me of children in Latin America I had encountered through my expressive sandwork projects, who live in extreme social crisis situations. Occasionally a smile will flit across the faces of such children, and when it does, it goes right through you. It is the children who were not fortunate enough to grow up in line with their level of development but who, so I assume, nevertheless experienced a certain degree of love from an adult or adults, who can smile in this particular way. It instantly moves one to tears although one couldn't say why. This is what happened to me when U. glanced at me at the beginning of the second session. But let us proceed step by step and not head over heels, even if U. was thrown head over heels into the world and has by no means already recovered from the multiple traumas this caused him.

The adoptive parents brought the boy to therapy because his outbursts of rage were becoming more frequent. He would become enraged if he found something unjust, when he was reprimanded, or when, for example, he had to leave home for his afternoon classes. He would often run out of the room, screaming loudly, only to return submissively a few minutes later, asking repeatedly, almost compulsively, for forgiveness. The parents were also concerned for the younger siblings, with whom U. was becoming more rough. When his brothers and sister were playing around, he would join in, but his parents described that his body would remain stiff as a board. U. suffered from nightmares, and he would often begin to cough in his sleep. After a while the coughing would become so bad that U. would vomit, without waking up. The boy never asked for a hug, in fact he mostly rejected them. Only when his father massaged his back did U. relax a little. The parents felt that U. was not listening to them when they spoke to him, and they bemoaned that he was like a bottomless barrel, that the infinite attention and love he received seemed to fall into nothingness. What is more, his mother emphasised, he could really tyrannise his younger siblings. The parents showed me photos of their family with the three completely healthy, adventurous children next to their parents, and U., the eldest, standing a few steps away with slumped shoulders as if he didn't even belong in the scene. The parents were open-minded and understanding, but they were also often at their wits' end. "I have a question," said the father, a practically minded man doing his best to understand his adopted son. "Couldn't this just be U.'s character and we should try to accept him exactly as he is?" I responded, "to a certain degree, for sure. To a larger degree, however, no child is born with these behaviours; they must be developed in order to survive extreme adversity."

First session:

As I mentioned earlier, U. had signalled to me with his body language that he would bear no intervention on my part whatsoever. Each of my comments or questions sent a wave of tension through his body, a huge question mark appearing in his pained little face as he desperately tried to understand what I meant, and knowing at the same time that whatever it was, it would have no meaning to him. When, after a few minutes, I finally said, "All right, now I'm going to stop with these questions, and you can play in peace," his body began to relax, and he explored the room with his gaze. He approached the shelves with the miniature figures. U. made the impression of having a rich inner life but also of residing on another planet. After some time of this silent togetherness, I felt that I, along with the sandtray and miniature figures, had landed on his planet and now had to submit to his strict rules. Something in his nature was excessive and forceful, and I caught myself reacting obediently. U.'s primary relationship pattern must have been marked by absence because it appeared that he could only really access his inner needs when he was alone. And so, I followed his actions with my gaze, although U. was currently doing nothing but standing rooted to the spot in front of the sector on the shelf with all the ships and boats. He regarded them for a long time, as if in trance. He touched one ship very cautiously and then another, as though afraid they might break. Then he took a wooden sailing ship in his hand, studied it from every angle, and placed it determinedly in the sandtray. At once, the sand turned into vast, grey ocean. It was frightening to suddenly see so much water and rolling crests of waves. U. crouched so that he had the sandtray at eye level and began to let the little ship glide across it in slow motion. It appeared fragile and hopelessly exposed to the elements. U. was absolutely concentrated, almost hypnotised – or was is dissociated? A bomb could hit the house, I thought, and he wouldn't notice. U. had now fetched more ships, and they each made their rounds, led by his hands. But then, almost imperceptibly, one ship began to sink. It had first tipped a little to one side and was now being drawn down slowly, as if by an undertow. U could see that I had noticed, and so I risked a comment: "Oh, the ship is sinking now." U. nodded. The ship kept sinking slowly until even the uppermost tip of the mast had disappeared under the surface and one couldn't even have said where exactly the ship had sunk. Then another ship approached from far away and began a long and tedious rescue manoeuvre. First, a diver searched in vain for the sunken ship. Then it was finally located and gradually pulled out of the water. One after

91

another, the sails billowed once more. Saved! The great sense of relief did not need to be articulated; a spontaneous, liberating sigh from both of us said it all. Our bodies were communicating, and it felt as though the verbal censorship U. had imposed on me remained one of the conditions. This scene was repeated. A different ship capsized and was pulled downwards in the same eerie manner as before; this time the rescue ship arrived sooner and the manoeuvre was completed more swiftly. "This ship was rescued too," I said. The fact that U. was facing me showed me that it was important to him that I understood, and I felt that he now might accept a few words. But it still appeared essential that I addressed him verbally only on the level of play, as if there were no reality outside of play. This catering to his unspoken needs brings to mind the state of reverie in early infancy. It allowed U. to focus on himself and on his ideas in the presence of another person, and to continue his play undisturbed. Thus, in the first minutes of his first session, he had already managed to depict content that was closely related to an original trauma. Depictions of accidents and rescue manoeuvres were repeated and varied over all of the following sessions. If I was unsure that I had understood everything correctly, I expressed a describing hypothesis which U., solely responsible for script and direction of all occurrences, could either accept or reject. This way he always felt maximally self-effective but also accompanied, and his inner security grew further and further.

I interpret this first act of his play, ships sinking and being rescued, as the portrayal of a dramatic, extremely threatening start to life, and also as a description of his current situation: no solid ground beneath his feet, going through life as if adrift in the open ocean, exposed to great mood swings and emotional storms, threatened to be pulled down by an undertow of depression but so far always being rescued again. U. continued to stage ships sinking in slow motion and subsequently being rescued, and there were already variations in this sequence. This is remarkable for the first sandplay scene in the first session. There were people sitting on the boats, then falling overboard almost unnoticed and disappearing into the water, only to be rescued again in complicated recovery missions. After about twenty minutes, U. cleared away the ships. One could see how confidently he already moved through the room and how he had appropriated the offer of play. Now he fetched miniatures of trees and animals. A forest was set up and both carnivores and herbivores placed in groups in the landscape. It was clear that the sand now represented solid ground and no longer water. I saw this as progress. Then – it happened so fast, I almost missed it – an elk was bitten by a cheetah and was left lying on the ground, wounded. I noticed U.'s emotion and tried to keep my comment as neutral as possible, while also indicating to him that I had witnessed the drama: "The cheetah bit the elk." He responded, "Yes, it is wounded and has hidden behind a bush." U. had talked to me for the first time. Because U.'s emotions were already clearly visible and palpable to me, I had tried, remaining on the level of play, merely to repeat the action: "The cheetah bit the elk." "Yes, it is wounded..." had been the answer, and there was satisfaction in U.'s tone, as if to say, "So you understood." Had I instead said, "The poor elk!" this would only have addressed one of many emotions that could possibly be relevant to U. In that moment it could just as well have been more important for U. to feel the cheetah's lust to bite rather than the elk's pain. And had I tried to arouse his empathy for the elk before he was ready, our emotional perceptions would have remained polarised: U. identifying with the aggressive cheetah, and I empathising with the elk. In this case, however, an interest for the wounded elk, who had "hidden in the bushes," had come from U. himself. He could just as well have said, "and now the cheetah is going to find another animal to bite."

I see this as a further step of progress towards empathic self-perception rather than dissociation. It goes without saying that the therapist perceives and must try to endure the dichotomic tension that builds up in play, without seeking to influence the direction. The therapist waits and sees where the child decides to take the plot next. It is interesting to see that children themselves mostly do not know how the course of play is going to continue. One thing leads to another and children learn to rely on an unconscious flow of images, a condition for every creative process.

A little while later, U. cleared away this scene as well and began to set up soldiers. Attacking and being attacked, confrontational dispute appeared to be the next topic. U. did this very accurately and proudly, as though he were now wholly in his element. Two equally powerful armies stood opposite each other. He told me he would like to show this scene to his father, who was waiting for him in the waiting room. Our first session ended and it felt to me as though U. had completed at least a few different therapy sessions in just that one hour. Between the sinking ships and the armies lining up in orderly fashion for combat he had achieved a good deal of self-determination.

The parents reported that the boy was like a new person in that first week after beginning therapy: happy, active, and communicative. He had told his brothers and sister every little detail of what he had played in the sand.

Second session:

A shy smile, somewhere between joyful expectation and incredulity, moved me deeply as I opened the door to the waiting room. And then he had already slipped past me and into the practice while I was still saying hello to his mother. In that moment of renewed encounter, his psychophysical system must have intuitively grasped that something "unheard of" would repeat itself again today: he would be allowed to pursue his own imaginations, undisturbed; to follow only his inner laws, some of them not even yet known to him; he would be allowed to search for his very own equilibrium without interference from the outside world, but in the company of an empathic adult. When he saw me again, sheer joy sparkled in his eyes at this prospect, this opportunity to exist just as he was; as if he knew that he would be able to use that one hour to catch up on something which had almost been smashed completely in the first months of his life history. I believe the fact that this fleeting smile touched me so immediately shows how deeply rooted this offer of communication is. My own psycho-somatic system reacted as if a baby had smiled at me for the first time in its life.

U. was eager to play with the soldiers again that day. Naturally, he had already set up both armies last session but had run out of time to play with them. But now he was uncertain and couldn't quite remember how he had placed the soldiers last time. He wanted the scene to be exactly the same as before. In other words, he was afraid that he might no longer be able to access his own ability to play. This is typical of children with dissociative tendencies because they can't rely on their own abilities. One day they find mental calculations the easiest thing and are proud of themselves, the next day it is as if everything had been wiped away. Memory and other cognitive abilities are extremely sensitive to disturbances. They can be obstructed in the long term by various factors, and they hinge on a person's overall mood. This led U. to want to hold on to the same patterns in play. The father had described U.'s play at home as frequently monotonous. He would, for example, drop marbles from different heights and observe how far they rolled. I helped U. find the same figures from his last session, but I also tried to make it clear that it could still be meaningful play, even if it was not exactly the same as last time. Thus, on the one hand, I accepted his concerns, and, on the other hand, I assured him of a free and protected space (everything is here for you and you can use it all again just as you need it; nobody expects you to adjust to anything). This allowed him to think, "even if the figures aren't exactly the same as last time, I might still feel the same way about them." And he was able to experience first-hand that it doesn't necessarily take a specific object or action to avert a threatening depressive mood. Eventually U. took a few of the soldiers from last time and a few new ones. He positioned the two armies, which were clearly defined, so he explained to me, as good and bad.

Compared to the previous session, U. was outright talkative, but also somewhat hectic, as if he were afraid that the miracle of the last session would not repeat itself and that everything good he had gained would disappear before his eyes, a common feeling in adopted children.

Once all the soldiers were in position, U. explained to me, almost as if to apologise for something that might appear childish, "At home I always do like this when they shoot." He followed the line of fire from one soldier to an opposing soldier, where it was then revealed if the latter was hit, wounded or killed. He erected fortifications on both sides with damp sand, and then the soldiers began to fight each other in pairs. He followed the lines of fire with immense concentration and effort.

It was fascinating, but just as strenuous, to watch. The free and protected space allowed U. moments of deep regression, which were then followed by progressive sequences. His emotional age changed many times during the session, and he was able to try himself in many different situations, both in his identification with the portrayed figures and in his relationship with the therapist. At the conclusion of this scene, after many soldiers had fallen on both sides, his face glowed with satisfaction, and he said, "The good ones won."

Next, he wanted to set up another scene of war. He placed the armies in a similar fashion and the scene began once more. Again, I could see his exertion and feel my own. Time dragged on, that day's session appearing to last for ever. I didn't mind because U. needed time. Once he was finished, he reached the same relieved conclusion: the good ones won. It was absolutely clear that the outcome of these confrontations was not foreseeable for U. He had not consciously decided who would win. It just happened to be the good side. The fact that it was important for U. to discern between good and bad likely meant that he perceived himself as very bad, something that applies to a lot of children who struggle with aggression.

Next, U. said he wanted to play something else. He fetched trees – two bare ones and a few green ones – and two tigers and an elk. "So he's going to pick up a theme from the first session," I thought to myself. He found the little white doves and placed them very patiently on the branches. Then the action commenced. The tiger seized the elk, threw it to the ground, and wanted to start eating it. The elk managed to escape, limping, and hid behind the trees. U. looked up at me, so I said, "The tiger attacked the elk and the elk ran away." "Yes," he answered, like a director contemplating the possible continuation of the plot. "The tiger bit it." He said it with concern and compassion in his voice. The fact that I in my unspoken thoughts and emotions associated the elk's wounding with everything that I knew about U.'s life, implicitly created an atmosphere – a psychic field – in which the suffering, the fear, the rage, the helplessness, but also the ability to save himself were all present, were supported by me, and could therefore be experienced more consciously by U. He was able to enter into inner resonance with whichever emotion he most needed in the moment to process the wounds of his past.

I trusted that U. would signal how much he wanted to share, what and when, and whether he wanted my reaction. As long as U. was depicting a dramatic scene in his play and was clearly emotionally captured by it, I knew that psychological processing was at work. When a therapist accepts the relationship modality defined by the child, it allows the child to share feelings that are still unknown even to itself. Until then, these feelings may only ever have overcome the child as inner restlessness, agitation, or paralysis, but the child will gradually learn to differentiate them and recognise them as its own.

Conversations with U. and his adoptive mother:

At the beginning of the third therapy session, I invited U.'s mother, who had accompanied him, into the therapy room for a talk. U. sat on his mother's lap. I had already told the parents in our precursory conversations about the importance of free, symbolic play for self-reflection, emotional differentiation and self-regulation, and the processing of current conflicts and past traumas. The mother had told me that U.'s younger siblings were ahead of him in their development and were often bored by his repetitive play habits. At the same time, U. would become angry and violent if his brothers and sister even dared come near his Lego constructions. I had told them it would be important for U. to have his own play corner, where his toys could be used only by him. This proved difficult to realise in daily family life. U. complained that his siblings always "smashed and destroyed" everything, while his mother tried to point out that they only occasionally disassembled his Lego constructions. It was clear that U. found it difficult to see continuity in creation and destruction, re-creation and re-destruction. As is common for so many people who have suffered traumas, he perceived destruction as final. In U.'s presence, I had told his parents that his siblings' actions felt like destruction and devastation to U., but that we would find ways to change this. U. would also have fits of rage because he didn't want to go back to school for afternoon classes. Losing time at play was an utter horror to him. And rightly so, as a matter of fact. Symbolic play was, at that moment, his main way to make new experiences. His parents, on the other hand, were concerned that so much childlike play would lead to withdrawal in a ten-year-old. Using emotion cards, we explored together how U. and his mother felt when it came to the matter of homework. He felt anger and a tendency to withdraw, she felt distraught, powerless, and angry. She wanted to be more cheerful, and he wanted to be calmer and more confident. During one of these sessions, the mother asked me with U. sitting on her lap if I thought that U. had been listening to her because he hadn't answered her question. We had just been speaking about his difficulties with homework. I replied that I assumed U. had listened, even if he didn't answer, but that we could just ask him. "Yes," came his answer, he had been listening. But then why hadn't he responded to his mother's question? "Because I didn't want to." This was a new statement, and I saw it as a decisive step. Perhaps for the first time in his life, U. was able to verbalise – without becoming angry – that he didn't want something. This led to a very helpful conversation because I was able to explain to U. that if he was silent, his mother believed he hadn't listened. If on the other hand he told her that he didn't want something, she would understand that and wouldn't be angry at him. He granted us a smile. The tendency not to listen often has to do with dissociative states that children needed to develop in their early childhoods for their psyche's survival. In U.'s case today, not listening appeared to have also become a habit of passive resistance: he understood very well what was being said, he just couldn't articulate that he didn't want what was being said. For the mother, this was an important step to better understanding U. She could now ask more precise questions: "Were you listening or don't you want to hear what we were just talking about?"

Already in the third session, a completely new play variation opened up. U. fetched houses and placed them in the sand with exact deliberation. He built roads and created different areas that were separated from each other but were not self-contained. There were at least five scenes depicting people (mostly families) spending leisure time together, for example at an ice skating rink. The organic composition of the whole image, the attention to detail, and perhaps the ice skating in particular, reminded me of a winter painting by Bruegel the Elder. The longer one looked at it, the more scenes one discovered, all of them related but each with its own narrative. It appeared as if U. was successfully sorting his different relationship experiences and emotional states, one by one. While all of the scenes were connected through paths and streets, the prison was the exception. For good reason, as U. explained: there were two men in there who had stolen something. The prison was quite spacious. I had the impression that U. was afraid of the two men. I was also struck by a sudden feeling of nausea and said, "They must be *really* bad." I could see relief in U.'s face that he had momentarily been able to banish everything fear-associated to one place, where it couldn't do any harm. There was a castle at the upper edge of the image. A father with a child in his arms and a mother lived there, U. explained. An ambulance stood next to the castle. U. only used fantasy figures in human and animal form. In terms of development, these figures correspond to the magical phase between five and nine years of age.

For U., this scene must have been about integrating his own positive life experiences in his adoptive family, about creating relationships between different inner domains and emotional states, and about autonomy and movement (the vehicles). The cars drove quietly and reliably (there were more accidents and rescue manoeuvres to come in the following sessions). The emphasis here was clearly on establishing relations, exploring, and recognising and re-treading paths that were free of hazards.

The fourth session brought a kind of summary of everything that had been achieved thus far, and a preview of the next phase. In this scene, the sandtray was divided into two large areas: water and ships in the left half (readers will recall the play sequence of the first session), and dry land with houses, roads, cars and people on the right. Again, he erected a prison. He continued to do so over many of the following sessions. This scene was a clear attempt to combine the two realms of land and water: a harbour and pier were added to the large area of water so that boats could dock, and towards the end of the session a restaurant was even added to the harbour, "so that the people could get something to eat." In the land half of the scene, the previous session's play was more or less repeated. There were houses, people, and connecting roads.

Occasionally a car lost control in the curve, only to be repaired by mechanics, who were on the spot very quickly.

The theme of "bad men in prison" was repeated again and again over the following sessions. The men would try to escape and to kill people. Once a woman was shot – a mother – and the men were brought back to prison. Some of them "became good", others remained bad. U. almost broke into a sweat when he was dealing with this issue, revealing how important it was for him that I see and follow all of this. I assumed that U. was processing incidents in these sessions that he had never consciously perceived but that were stored in his body memory: brutal violence and threats to his life. Over the same period, his parents reported that his fits of rage and dissociative moments had become less frequent, and that he was generally more cheerful.

During the fifth session, U. himself showed me something significant. Unprompted, he explained to me, "That big dinosaur there is the father of this one here." The fact that it was precisely a family relationship between two play figures that he wanted to explain to me (father and son) indicated that the basic conditions for the activation of a dialogical dimension (two instances can communicate) in his psyche had been met. This topic also corresponded well to his age: a ten-year-old boy becoming more clearly aware of his male identity, trying to follow his father's role model, and generally trying to understand the fatherly principle in the world. Despite all of his traumatic primary experiences, U. demonstrated very clearly that there was a vital side in him that was intensely focused, physiologically and psychologically, on reaching the next developmental level. It was during this phase that he once remarked during a session, when I had become distracted, "Aren't you writing this down?"

After five therapy sessions – the equivalent of one and a half months – I asked the parents "how things were going", and they told me about the following changes in U.'s behaviour at home. He now asked to be hugged and cuddled multiple times a day. He played with his brothers and sister more often, in part also because his play suggestions had become more interesting for the younger children. He showed more motivation to do his homework. In the previous week, he had lost control and become aggressive only once, and the short amount of time it took him to calm down again astounded the whole family.

These changes they described pertained to different behaviours. What they had fundamentally in common, however, was that U. had become more consciously aware of his physical and emotional needs and had learnt to rely on the fact that the adults would recognise these needs and – in part – fulfil them. U.'s therapy continued for another year, in which his progress regarding social behaviour was confirmed by his family, his teachers, and fellow students. My verbal interventions during the sessions never deviated from what I have described here: making certain I had seen and understood things correctly, and verbalising actions and incidents in play, when U. showed strong emotional involvement. U. was never bored or uncertain what he should play. This shows how great his urge to catch up on free, symbolic play must have been. On the other hand, since U. could now express himself better, his developmental deficits on a cognitive level became more apparent. I recommended individual sessions with a teacher using the Feuerstein method, which U. accepted willingly. U.'s treatment continued and soon brought a phase in which language and narration became ever more important.

FOURTH CHAPTER

Expressive Sandwork

We humans are social beings and need each other to maintain the equilibrium of our bodies and souls. Perhaps the soul is not just hidden inside us, perhaps it is precisely *between* us human beings that *soul develops.*

Expressive sandwork[7], the method I will introduce in the following, has to do with such an invisible band between people. Over the past 15 years, volunteer participants from different professional backgrounds have made expressive sandwork an efficient form of psychosocial aid for children suffering from neglect, violence, and abuse. Expressive sandwork takes place in parts of the world where psychological care is scarcely available: Chinese and Romanian orphanages, makeshift settlements in Africa and Latin America, and refugee accommodation in Malaysia, Germany, and Ukraine.

Hillman (From Mirror to Window: Curing Psychoanalysis of its Narcissism, 1989) wrote that it is time psychoanalysis attended to social problems. While analysts and their patients have spent

---

[7] I developed this method in cooperation with Jungian analysts from South Africa, Latin America, and China, based on the analytic psychology of C.G. Jung and building upon the sandplay methods of Margaret Lowenfeld and Dora Kalff. See Pattis Zoja (2011).

enough time regarding themselves in mirrors, Hillman writes, all around them a society in need is waiting. Picking up on Hillman's statement today, we could say that it has become necessary to move not just from the mirror to the window but from the window to the door. Faced with worldwide migration phenomena, many psychotherapists across the world are prepared to open their private practices and to rethink their individual spheres of action and theoretical concepts. This brings to mind Freud's idea to make free therapy sessions available to people in need who could not afford psychoanalytical treatment. This social vision of psycho-analysis was realised with the foundation of the "free clinics" in Vienna and Berlin, which operated between 1920 and 1933 until they were abolished by the Nazi regime. Almost 100 years on, expressive sandwork sees itself as a small contribution to this vision in a world that has changed considerably. The important contributions of psychology and psychoanalysis over the past 100 years have helped us expand our capacity to perceive reality, and to uncover what mostly remains invisible around us. They have allowed our psyches to merge experiences from our individual unconscious and from the collective unconscious. Thanks to this development, which has affected our individual consciousness, one could even say that, recently, a new level of experience has gradually become visible: the collective consciousness. This means that our individual consciousness also realises that we are part of a collective that influences us, and that we, with every slightest action, influence in turn. Each of us is an individual consciousness, but also part of a system. I see expressive sandwork as an expression of the activation of this collective consciousness, with its origins in the "caring" environment of a human being.[8]

Expressive sandwork is a cross-cultural, non-verbal method revolving around the processing of traumatic experiences. It

---

[8] *Expressive Sandwork: An Experience Working with Columbian Vulnerable Population*, by Eva Pattis Zoja and Eduardo Carvallo, IAAP-Congress in Copenhagen 2013.

addresses a child's or adolescent's self-healing powers and consciously refrains from verbalising or interpreting the play action. Seen in this light, the method is a chance to become psychotherapeutically effective without being limited by language barriers. The aim is to allow the soul's inner experiences to be visualised with the help of a sandtray and different materials and play figures, and to process those same experiences through creative action.

Expressive sandwork rests upon three pillars. The first is the symbolic function that unfolds when a child depicts its inner world in the sand. The second is the bond between the child and the facilitator, which develops during the process and can restore the primary relationship. The third pillar is formed by the group, which holds the (child-adult) dyad together like an alchemical container.

Furthermore, expressive sandwork combines two theoretical premisses that both emanate from a teleological point of view of psychological phenomena.

1. *The psyche's tendency towards self-regulation*, a concept influenced by C.G. Jung. This means that the psyche continuously produces spontaneous, emotionally loaded images and entire image processes with the purpose of counteracting existing mental and emotional imbalances. We adults know such visual processes from our dreams. In children, there is also imaginative play.

2. John Bowlby (1969), on the other hand, illustrated the absolute significance of the *primary relationship* between mother and child for the development of internal working models of our togetherness with other people.

If it is true that the psyche is able to "regulate itself", then it follows our biological needs as mammals that this type of regulation would be aligned towards attachment and relationship. We need others in order to develop. We could also say that *development* and *relationship* are the two great motivating factors of our human existence. This leads us to one of the central factors of expressive sandwork's effectiveness. It takes place in a group. The fact that children and adults share a large room creates a feeling of security (i.e. reducing fear), which in turn promotes explorative play. Thus, a very inhibited child, for example, can afford to do nothing at first and can just stand and watch what the others are doing for a few sessions. The group signals the child non-verbally that nothing else is expected. This offers the child an external "safe place," which is the precondition for self-regulating processes to take place in the psyche. These processes, meanwhile, gradually create an internal safe place, which in turn is the precondition for processing trauma. It may even be the case that collective traumas, such as we have seen in war zones, are *best* healed through and in a group setting. When a village community is massacred – as happened in Colombia, for example, during the fifty-year armed conflict between government troops, paramilitaries, and guerrilla fighters – not only is every individual survivor's psyche injured to the core, the community of individuals, the collective soul, is also injured. Each individual's trust in human togetherness is broken. We shall see how this healing process of an entire community is depicted by children in sandplay again and again: first destruction, then healing through collective meals and celebrations, as if children knew that rituals were important.

When we speak of a traumatic experience, we usually mean something that exceeds what we are capable of processing psychologically. Instead, the psyche produces ways of perceiving the world that protect against renewed injury (e.g. apathy). The downside is that, from then on, the individual will live life "on low flame" as far as relationships and emotions are concerned: options for new experiences are extremely limited, and it is precisely the situations where self-efficacy could be tested that are avoided – in children this pertains, above all, to imaginative play. This creates a vicious circle. Despite all of this, there is an archetypically rooted readiness of the psyche to make new relationship experiences. In other words, *because* we are social beings, something deep inside us never stops searching for an "other". Expressive sandwork makes use of this self-regulating function of the psyche that is oriented towards attachment. Children play in a sandtray without any instructions whatsoever. Two months later, their improved social competence is noticeable to their parents or educators. Nobody showed them how to achieve greater self-confidence. Nobody taught them that it is better to cooperate than to steal each other's toys. So where did they learn this? During their own play in the sandtray in the presence of a reference figure. Three factors are required, which must remain constant over a period of at least three months: the offer of imaginative play, the presence of an unchanging adult for each child, and the group.

In practice, the situation is as follows: A group of children and adults is assembled in a large room, each child sits or stands at a sandtray, busy creating its own world, and an adult sits alongside each sandtray. The room is silent. Countless miniature figures and objects are set up in the middle of the room, sorted by category: people, animals, houses, cars, trees, shells, marbles. Again and again, the children move back and forth between the play material and their sandtrays, fetching a particular little animal, soldiers, building blocks, or toy cars. The children do not disturb each other, all apparently preoccupied with their own imaginations. Some of the adults sitting next to the sandtrays are so discreet, one hardly notices them. If one looks more closely, however, one occasionally sees their expressions changing unexpectedly, revealing their deep involvement. A very special psychic space is created during the sessions between each child and "his" or "her" adult. If there is any speaking at all, then only at a level that does not disturb the others. Most of the communication takes place through body language, especially eye contact. Between twelve and twenty weekly sessions are offered, each lasting an hour. Children can also finish and leave the room sooner, if they wish, while the other children continue playing.

Now, what do the adults do, who, as we have heard, do not necessarily have any psychological training? Or, more to the point, what *don't* they do? They do not ask questions and do not comment. They try to observe what is happening in the play sequence, what emotional effect it is having on the child, and what effect on themselves. Of course, they also notice changes in the *contents* of play. If a number of past sessions were marked by confrontations and fighting in the sand, a facilitator may well think to herself, "Here we go again..." before the next session. But if she then sees the child carrying a handful of football players to the sandtray instead of soldiers, a referee, and two goals, she will likely be astounded. She will not only take mental note that the conflict appears to have shifted to a new level: since she herself had found herself in a war zone for session after session, as it were, she might well breathe a deep sigh of relief.

But how is this play related to the issue of attachment? Here is an example to illustrate. A boy has shown anxious-avoidant attachment since early childhood and is now offered the opportunity to do expressive sandwork. First of all, he is overjoyed with all of the play material and at having his own sandtray! But he doesn't know what to think about this empathic adult who appears to be "part of the package." "She should just leave me in peace," his body language appears to say. In the first session, the child might even begin to play with his back turned to the adult. Meanwhile, inside the sandtray, this avoidance is also depicted with the help of the play figures; but so is, very cautiously, a desire for attachment. This needs to be tested slowly and carefully. A child might place a mother pig and her piglets in the sand, then a mother horse and her foals, and also an infant child and a dog watching and apparently protecting it. During play, children are thoroughly preoccupied with "effecting things by themselves," frequently things they could never have effectuated in real life in their often hostile environments. This promotes confidence in themselves and in the world. And then, at some point during play, a quick, casual glance is cast in the direction of the adult: "Is she actually watching what I'm doing?" And then again, a little later, almost involuntarily. "Oh, now I've gone and collapsed the tunnel I've been working on for so long!" The adult *was* watching and shared the experience of the tunnel collapsing. Gradually, the adult's presence will be "used" emotionally by the child, in the very intensity that the child requires at the time. The child itself can regulate the level at which it would like to test attachment: on the symbolic level in play, or on a concrete level. One can almost watch as the two levels spur each other on. Play becomes more intense *because* an adult is present, and because play becomes more intense and emotionally challenging, the adult will be drawn in more closely. The child looks at the adult more frequently, play becomes more differentiated, and the shared experience becomes stronger, much like healthy attunement during infancy. Together the two sides create a pre-lingual, active form of *togetherness.* And this altogether new form of togetherness, *never before experienced* for some children, will establish itself in the psyche as a new internal working model in the sense of Bowlby (1969).

Expressive sandwork offers countless examples of this being possible in childhood and far into puberty. If children are only allowed to play long enough and regularly enough in this way, then all phases of a healthy development will be spontaneously recreated in play.

These phases can be read in the play sequences again and again: feeding, eating, caring, even "playing" is played in the sand. And then, finding friends, fighting, conquering, owning, sharing, etc. An inner wealth of experience and emotions is created from which children can then dare to confront traumatic experiences. A child's psyche itself knows *when* the time is right.

Regarding attachment theory, we could also ask ourselves: how can it be that models of relationship acquired early in life can be altered through imaginative play, of all things? Can a child's psyche really produce an alternative to the style of attachment developed in earliest childhood?

D. Winnicott's (1971) description of the transitional object is helpful in this case. To a little child, a comfort blanket is a functional dialogue partner on a pre-lingual level, and is expression of a relationship function. Another concept is provided by Panksepp (1998), who has studied play behaviour in mammals for the past twenty years. Panksepp showed that play not only fulfils an affect-regulating function. Its primary purpose is the development of social competence. The unfortunate, play-deprived rats with which he worked showed general deficiencies in their development, but their social incompetence was particularly striking. Thus, one of the main functions of the play system is learning about relation-ships. Panksepp only studied rough and tumble play in animals and children. Since the human brain, however, is a symbolic organ (his own words) and since humans are cultural beings, it is safe to say that learning about relationships and making up for relationship deficits takes place *precisely* on a metaphoric, imaginative, and symbolic level in humans. And, in children, this level is play. Fortunately, we humans are not just trapped in irreversible biological imprinting, like Konrad Lorenz's geese. What was imprinted on us in earliest childhood can be altered *precisely* because we are able to represent and experience things *figuratively*. Ill-fated primary relationships can be "repaired" because a symbol-producing function of the psyche continuously and autonomously tries to achieve precisely what has been so unsuccessful thus far. This happens spontaneously in childhood through play. But play alone is not enough, nor is the offer of relationship alone. It takes both. Play points the way in this process; it defines content, speed, and rhythm. A sensitive offer of relationship *only* has a healing effect in those moments when children themselves sought it: the rest of the time is spent waiting for those precise moments.

In summary, we could say of expressive sandwork: it is a system consisting of a number of subsystems. The following example illustrates how this structure of systems can be expressed in a sandtray by a child. The creator of this sand image was a fourteen-year old girl. The main theme of this girl's expressive sandwork was nourishment and care. We can see nurses and doctors, each caring for a baby in a pushchair. Milk bottles have been carefully arranged in the middle of a round table. The number of pairs (nurses and babies) corresponds exactly to the number of children and adults in the project. Aside from the symbolic content (the mandala-like form in the middle of the table), the group dynamic is portrayed in realistic detail, revealing a deep trust in the fact that all individuals will find their place and will be cared for and respected. The twelve dyads form a secure container. The energies resonating in such a group are multiplied, as is the stimulating effect on the psycho-somatic systems of all participants, be they children or adults.

When a child plays motherly care, this is not an act of com-pensation (the child does not do this *because* it received too little such care); it is an expression of a caring function becoming activated *in* the child's psyche itself. To use neuroscientist Jaak Panksepp's (1998) concepts, one could say that, among the many motivational biological systems on a neuronal level, the child's CARE system has been turned on. And this has an effect on the psyche's health. The same is true for many sand images depicting, for example, nature as the predominant theme, harmony among animals, or figures caring for each other.

During the sessions, a "psychic space" develops between facilitator and child, which shields them, to a certain degree, from their surroundings. The constancy of the elements – room, sand-tray, facilitator – is essential to foster an atmosphere of trust throughout the entire process. Slowly but surely, bridges are built between the two, and also, on another level, between everyone participating in this process. The sessions require a large room so that the play material and sandtrays can be properly set up. The children are offered at least twelve weekly sessions of an hour each with the same volunteer facilitator. Aside from this visible part of the process, there is often also a more intimate, invisible process, the development of the attachment between volunteer facilitator and child described above. Perhaps the strength of this relationship derives precisely from a deep, often neglected desire to win back and activate ritual spaces of connectedness with others.

In the following, I would like to give the account of a primary school teacher from Romania, who took on the role of group facilitator for the entire group during a sandwork project Here is the teacher's description:

"During this project, I will 'only' be a group facilitator for the entire group. The other volunteer facilitators will each get to work with a single child," I had told myself. But the experience turned out different than expected, and I was happy for my role. I was completely and utterly involved – physically, intellectually, and emotionally. I saw the adult-child duo with my eyes and my heart, and I was flooded with emotions that I was only gradually able to differentiate. I grew along with these pairs. Most of them were quite similar. It wasn't easy. A few nights in a row, I dreamt I was digging in the sand. At one point, I was tired and shivered with cold. This was after a session more or less midway through the project. The atmosphere was heavy. I feel pain in my arms and shoulders. I feel burdened. I hear a child thumping on the sand. The sound drones in my ears. I can only hear that one sound. My whole body aches. Maybe these children feel a similar pain. I look into the volunteers' faces and recognise their pain as well. All of us can feel this pain. At the end of the session, the child who was pounding the sand looks up at me. His expression is peaceful. He appears to have left all of his pain in the sand, and I understand that.

The Setup of the Expressive Sandwork System

The children

People in responsible positions select the children who are to take part in expressive sandwork. These are mostly school teachers, social workers from organisations (governmental or non-governmental) working with the local population, or people with a connection to the church community. We are careful not to define specific criteria for selecting the children. Every child that feels like "playing with sand" can participate. Even without a formal selection procedure, we have observed that those responsible in the communities do appear to make a selection based on intuition and common sense. Mostly, the emphasis is on heterogeneity. This can lead to strong, healthy children working right next to problematic children, which makes for intense group-dynamic effects. To use a metaphor from physics, through resonance, the vibrations of the different individuals within the group (children and adults) tend to combine to a "group vibration", and this, in turn, tends towards harmony. Perhaps it is for this reason and because the children have "their own adults" all to themselves in each session, that the children find it easy to follow the few rules in place: work alone; work in silence; when speaking is necessary, only speak to your own adult; do not disturb the others; do not disperse sand outside of the sandtray.

The play material

A further issue is the selection of play material. It must offer enough scope to process traumatic experiences. This is why war material such as tanks, soldiers, and weapons must also be provided, as must figures that represent violence and danger. Another point requiring consideration is the issue of values. Faced with different religious affiliations in particular, the symbolic objects and figures provided must allow for a value-neutral depiction of transcendent references. The items on offer range from natural materials, small technical parts such as screws, nails, and rails, to all sorts of human play figures. Furthermore, there are animals of every kind, plants, but also cars, aeroplanes, boats, and ships. As in sandplay therapy, the aim is to provide as broad a spectrum as possible, corresponding to the children's horizon of experience. Unlike sandplay therapy, however, the selection of different play figures need not be as large in expressive sandwork. Instead, there should definitely be "enough of the same," so that the children can be assured of finding the same materials they require for their images, each session.

The volunteers

The volunteer facilitators undergo an extensive selection procedure at the outset of each project. They have different professional backgrounds, such as teachers, social workers, pensioners, artists, students, psychologists, and psychotherapists. The decisive criteria for selection are their capacity to regulate and reflect their own emotions and their reliability. Since each child works with one specific facilitator, there is no substitution and the facilitators must guarantee their presence during each session and each meeting throughout the entire process. The facilitators receive a brief but thorough introduction and continued supervision throughout the project. An essential element of this training procedure is two sessions of hands-on experience with sandplay. The adults work in pairs and take turns playing the roles of actor and observer. It goes without saying that each child's unconscious elicits an intense emotional reaction in the facilitator's psyche. Therefore, the whole group and each individual facilitator is supported throughout the entire process by the project leader. There are intervision sessions, where the facilitators can talk about their experiences in the sessions, about emotional impact, doubts, fears, and concerns. There could be moments when the facilitator feels an urge to act, for example, to give the child a present or to visit the child's family at home. Such reactions require very cautious reflection and therapeutic containment. For this reason alone, aside from a number of practical ones, attendance of the intervision sessions in small groups is a "conditio sine qua non" of expressive sandwork. The alchemical reaction between facilitator and child is triggered in the very first minutes of their coming together. We do not assign children to facilitators or vice versa. In the first session, each child "selects" an adult with whom he or she will work throughout the entire process. The adults are already in the room and seated next to the sandtrays when the children enter the room together. Before coming into the room, the children are merely told to "just choose a sandtray." But of course, in those few minutes, they will also have "chosen" the adult sitting next to the sandtray. In our opinion, this selection process is based on the "tele" function described by Jacob Levy Moreno. We rely on the fact that the attachment between child and facilitator-to-be is a bi-directional process. We have long since stopped marvelling at synchronicities in the dynamics between child and facilitator: be they physical similarities or a "coagulation" of elements that had existed in the unconscious realm and gradually became conscious as the accompanying process unfolded. Among many issues, we have encountered something during the intervision talks that we call the "empty sandtray syndrome." It is easy to imagine how frustrating it must be for a facilitator if his or her child misses one or multiple sessions and the sandtray remains empty, while the other children are happily at work.

The parents

We strive to involve the parents in all sandwork projects. We offer a parent meeting at the beginning and at the end of a project. Furthermore, parents can approach the project leaders throughout the duration of the project if they have questions or would like to communicate anything.

The facilitator's attitude towards the parents is much like it is towards a child during a session: listening attentively without giving advice, valuing their perception, and appreciating their role as parents. Very soon, even anxious, abusive, and apathetic parents learn, non-verbally, a little bit of the facilitator's calm, accepting and respectful attitude towards the children. They learn to perceive a new quality that they themselves may never have experienced. The parents often notice how their child may have changed during and after a project, and they ask emphatically if the child's brother or sister could take part next time. The parents, however, are not allowed to attend the sessions themselves, and they never get to see the children's sand images.

FIFTH CHAPTER

Processing Trauma after Displacement in Colombia

Example 1

A., a nine-year-old girl from the north of Colombia, witnessed an armed attack on her village. She saw people lose their lives, including small children. Her own family was spared, but the leader of the guerrilla troops offered her father money if he would surrender his daughter to be trained as a guerrilla fighter. That same night her family fled to Bogotá and had since lived in a suburb known as *el Bronx*, where crime and drug and weapons trafficking are part of everyday life.

A. was anxious and suffered from poor sleep. Over the course of multiple sessions of expressive sandwork, A. made sand images depicting a peaceful world where people and animals lived together and children were each provided with their own bottle of milk, sitting on little chairs, watched over by adults or pets. There was also a little lake with ducks, and sheep grazing in a round paddock. These depictions were repeated with slight variations and different arrangements, but the atmosphere was always calm and harmonious. The child's facilitator had already begun to wonder if sandwork would prove to be the right medium for the girl because there was no sign whatsoever of anything difficult in her images. Then came the sixth session and, with it, a sudden change. A. had carefully covered all of the sand's surface with pink tulle fabric, before hectically placing armoured vehicles, soldiers, bombs, and weapons. The facilitator felt a sudden fear, almost panic, creeping up inside him. War. Perhaps the pink tulle was an attempt to soften the horror of the scene at least a little bit. Two soldiers were fighting each other in a jeep. Others were already shot. The whole lower part of the image showed rows of bombs.

Then A. placed the same little chairs in which the children had sat in previous scenes, each with their own bottle of milk. Only this time the chairs were empty. The facilitator felt a choking sensation when he saw these chairs. It reminded him that A. had witnessed infant children being killed. Not a word was spoken between the two.

After a while, A. began to work in the upper right corner. She had fetched a well and flowers from the collection of toys. In stark contrast to the scene of war, she now placed the well in this corner, as well as two cats, water, and flowers - a place of resilience.

There followed a number of sessions in which scenes of violence alternated with scenes of peaceful togetherness and shared meals, until, eventually, the latter prevailed. Today, the child is doing well. Self-regulation of the psyche also means that A. knew of her own accord when and how the traumatic experience was best depicted and processed.

Project leaders in Colombia have been able to observe how heavily traumatised children will always also depict resilience alongside the trauma-related content, provided they can play long enough under the conditions described, and provided there is an advance of trust in the symbolic process. Slowly but surely, it is this resilience that gains ground in the children's lives. As mentioned before, the adult's function in all of this is none other than being an emotional resonator, something for which most people are naturally talented. This is what makes volunteer facilitators so effective.

Example 2

Sandwork always encounters limitations whenever the free and protected space cannot be ensured. This is the case when the child's environment is not safe for the duration of the therapeutic process. We see this in active war zones or, in extreme cases, where abuse and maltreatment emanate from the family environment itself. We once encountered a six-year old boy in Latin America whose mother was being extorted by a drug cartel and saw herself forced to offer her son repeatedly for recordings of pornographic films. The boy's sandwork images showed a row of natural catastrophes, becoming greater and more destructive each time. In the end, it was the boy's behavioural problems outside of sandwork that led a social worker, who was not involved in the project itself, to call for his removal from his family environment and for him to be placed in a state-run home for children. The social worker refrained from notifying the police. She came from the same crime-saturated district and would have risked her own life and the lives of her family.

With the following example of an expressive sandwork process in a similar social environment in Latin America, I would like to illustrate the fine line between protected and unprotected space with which project leaders frequently have to cope.

Expressive sandwork not only helped this six-year old girl come to terms with a great burden, it also had a positive effect on the families of her neighbourhood because it allowed them to discover a new level of solidarity. From the first session, the facilitator realised that the little girl was expressing the great psychological burden from which she suffered. She piled a vast number of play items into her sandtray, mainly kitchen items and food but also insects, snakes, soldiers, and babies. She filled a few of the pans with sand and played "cooking". Suddenly she was filled with rage and knocked everything over, threw plates and pans on the ground, and even broke a few things intentionally. At the end of the session, she covered parts of the sandtray with a piece of cloth.

Amidst all this chaos, the volunteer was taken by one scene in particular. A reptile with its jaws opened wide approaching a baby in a pram, which the girl had covered with cloth. The volunteer remarked in her notes: "As I was clearing up after the session and lifted the cloth, I saw the reptile again and began to tremble. I felt cold... I was shocked and my whole body was shaking..."

This strong emotional reaction on the part of the volunteer and further similar scenes during the following sessions suggested that the child was in serious trouble, possibly suffering ongoing violence or sexual abuse. But as the facilitators are not psycho-therapists, and as, from an institutional point of view, they are also not authorised to suggest such a possibility without filing a complaint with the police, the matter was left in suspense for the moment. Expressive sandwork continued over a couple of months and the project included several meetings with the parents.

The little girl's representations became less and less chaotic. It seemed especially important to the child to distinguish clearly between good and evil. In the tenth session, an upper and a lower area were clearly demarcated. The girl erected a high straw barrier in the sand and moved to the side where the facilitator was sitting, where the good resided, as if she wanted to share this place with her and move as far away as possible from the realm of the bad. In this session, the facilitator perceived the child's strong sense of intimacy, as well as her search for trust.

Something quite similar occurred in the next session as well. The straw barrier was there once again, and the facilitator perceived a sense of closeness and intimacy, while the barrier provided them both protection from the outside world. The girl stayed by the volunteer's side while playing.

The day after this session, the little girl asked to talk to her teacher at school, making it clear that she had something important to tell her. The teacher agreed to listen, and the little girl told her that she was being sexually abused by one of her neighbours.

The teacher immediately initiated the medical, psychological, and legal procedures for such cases. The school doctor, the school psychologist, and the police all contacted the girl's parents. The accused, the father of a fourteen-year-old girl who was also participating in the project, fled the neighbourhood a few hours later. Fear had been lifted from the children of an entire apartment block.

The other children's parents were greatly alarmed, but they did not react in panic, and began to speak to their daughters over the following days. Two of the other girls reported similar incidents involving the same man.

In less favourable conditions, when a common enemy in a poverty-stricken and crime-ridden environment is identified, the revelation can easily unleash a reaction of hate and even more violence. In this case, however, the sandwork project had promoted solidarity among the affected families, especially among the women, and this united them. The problem was solved by uniting the social resources available in the community itself.

As the children were now safe, the mothers were able to face reality in a calm and rational way. This was particularly evident in the solidarity shown towards the wife and daughter of the abuser, who were terrified that they might suffer some kind of retribution. Regarding the abuser himself, on the other hand, it was tacit law in this slum that the other men would not wait for the police to find him. As to the little girl whose sandwork had initiated the whole episode, the sessions and her growing confidence in the facilitator had strengthened her own self-esteem and had given her the security that she would be listened to.

It must be pointed out that she had not gone to her facilitator, and had not requested intervention where it could not have been provided in such a direct way. The girl preserved her facilitator's role and, instead, sought help in the proper place, at school, in a public institution. She displayed incredible efficiency, probably because the necessary structure had already begun to emerge inside her. Although school and her teachers had been there long before, it was only through her sandwork experience that she gained the inner strength and self-esteem necessary to make use of these external resources. One thing is plain to see, here: without an activation of inner resources, even the most expensive interventions in socially weak milieus will hardly be effective.

Two years later, the girl, now eight years old, was able to take part in another project. In one of her last sand images it was plain to see that she had overcome her trauma. The straw mat leant over the peaceful scene in a protective manner. There was an opulently laid table, little sand cakes formed by the girl herself, a happy gathering of adults and children and many babies, each with a bottle of milk. At last, all of those involved could refresh and fortify themselves, and the children were cared for. The striking number of doctors and angels amongst the celebrating figures gave the scene a very special, ritual quality.

Example 3

The following account by Monica Pinilla Pineda, who has developed and advanced expressive sandwork with a team of Jungian analysts in Colombia since 2008, illustrates the long-term effect expressive sandwork can have on the lives of adolescents, even if they continue to live in the same problematic environments.

A thirteen-year-old girl lived in an outer district of Bogotá rife with trafficking of drugs and weapons. The social assistant, who had a huge number of children in similar situations to attend to, was alarmed because A. and a gang of other girls had become the female "mascots" of a gang of criminal adolescent boys, who conducted contract killings. The prospects for the future in such a situation and in this social context were usually a quick and irreversible decline into serious crime with a great risk of being murdered by an enemy gang. A. had gladly accepted the offer of sandplay. For an instant, her reserved expression had lightened, and her rough, aggressive manner had given way to a childlike curiosity, revealing a mountain of unsatisfied needs and desires.

A. was just reaching puberty, and others often called her a tomboy. Her hair was like a dry stick. Her mother was sexually abused by her own stepfather and became pregnant as a fifteen-year-old girl. When the baby was born, she was unable to love her, so the child was brought up by her grandmother. A. grew up on the outskirts of Bogotá, where few people knew about her story. Those who did tried to conceal it. Her mother moved to a different city with her two younger children, an eight-year-old boy and a six-month-old baby who were born to different men. She sometimes visited A. on weekends and gave the grandmother some money for the child's subsistence, but she could not handle spending much time with her daughter.

Her teachers were distressed by the girl's situation and did not know what to do. They found it impossible to work with her. She was aggressive and rude to others and often chose to isolate herself. A. and a gang of mid-teen girls were the "pet" girlfriends of a dangerous boys' gang. The boys dealt drugs and weapons and tried to assert themselves in the community through violence. One of A.'s teachers perceived the sadness behind her anger and invited her to take part in a series of expressive sandwork sessions.

When she came to her first session, A. was scared and maintained a distant attitude. I felt that my presence made her uneasy and could see that her upper lip was sweating. She turned her back to me and tried to hide what she was playing. Her entire attitude communicated that she preferred a certain distance to be kept. I took a step back. She looked a little calmer during the next sessions. She did not ask me for distance and let me accompany her and watch what she was doing. She kept creating the same scene, which she then covered with pieces of fabric so that it was hidden in the end. At one point, she placed the Virgin Mary holding the baby Jesus in what appeared to represent a nativity scene, which was then covered from view. She kept this up for a few sessions, playing and then covering the scene.

In the fifth session, she smiled at me for the first time upon entering the room. From this session on, she changed her play and started creating scenes that she then left uncovered. She started representing opposites that then became integrated, such as dangers in front of which she built protective spaces, or chaos near a sacred treasure. It was in the second to last session that she really surprised us. After entering the room, she kissed each of the volunteers on the cheek. In these last sessions, she depicted different aspects of the feminine and the masculine: women competing with each other and collaborating with each other and both protective and violent men. In the last scene, she carefully buried two men who had attacked and killed each other. Perhaps she also buried, here in these graves and before a witness, the sexual abuse she had suffered and was able to express her femininity and feel less vulnerable.

Once the project ended, A. left the girls' gang and her aggression seemed to lessen, while there were also noticeable changes in her previously dry hair and skin. Her grandmother reported an improvement in her performance at school. There were also changes in her relationship with her mother, who began to feel closer to her when she perceived how tender A. had become towards her baby brother. It appeared that this was also a new beginning in the mother-daughter relationship.

A Sandplay Session in Medellín, Colombia

Medellín, a city in the north of Colombia, is infamous for its crime associated with drugs and arms trade since the middle of the last century. The number of murders committed here by adolescents is still a sad record in all of Latin America. Over the past two decades, at least two architectural interventions by the city council have started to change the social climate. First, the city built cable cars (metrocable), which allow people from the high-lying favelas to find work down in the city and thus connected two social systems which had not been communicating. What is more, the city also built libraries in the favelas, offering children and adolescents a protected space where they could access a different world than the criminal environments they were exposed to every day.

If one takes such a cable car from the centre of Medellín, one reaches the altitude of Santo Domingo after about half an hour, a favela without infrastructure, where a huge, modern library towers over makeshift settlements like a fortress. In Santo Domingo, the most heavily armed gang gets to define the law. It has been years since the last law enforcement officers strolled the narrow streets that lead from the upper station of the cable car for about two kilometres along the mountainside to one of Santo Domingo's schools, where a session of expressive sandwork takes place every Saturday.

When the volunteer facilitators set off on this path, they wear white T-shirts bearing the word VOLONTARIO to signal that they are committed to social welfare and are unarmed. The way to the school leads past a number of little chapels with altars dedicated to the Virgin Mary. The young men bring their ammunition here to be blessed by the Mother of God before their big operations. It is the hope of everyone involved in this project that the prevailing attitude of silent complicity into which the population is forced will gradually change and that expressive sandwork might play a little

125

part in this process. Children who have taken part in a sandwork project will have experienced (at least for those three months) that safe places, reliable adults, and alternatives to fear and violence do exist. Above all, they will have experienced vividly that there is an inner world on which they can rely. Later, as adolescents, these children will be able to better defend their wishes and plans, and will hopefully be able to say "no", if they are ever drawn into the gang system. There are countless families in Santo Domingo, so-called "internal" refugees, who left their places of birth when their children were recruited by adolescent gangs, the boys to be trained as contract killers and the girls for prostitution.

Many of the children taking part in the Santo Domingo project have, or had, teenage parents: fathers were often already dead, killed in armed clashes, and the fifteen or sixteen-year-old mothers were left without support. Since they only have a short way to walk, the children arrive by themselves, sometimes with older siblings, and are usually on time for the sessions. It is a different story in situations where children live further away and depend on their parents to accompany them. These children regularly miss out on their sessions for the simple reason that there was nobody there to take them. It is difficult for these parents, who are still almost children themselves, who live close to the poverty line, and who are only tangentially aware of their children's everyday lives, to understand the purpose of such a project. For the children themselves, on the other hand, the sandtray with play figures exerts an irresistible fascination. It is as if children had some form of deeper knowledge that play could activate their very own, innate resources.

In the following, I would like to describe a session in Santo Domingo, based on the sandplay activities of some of the children. It was the second of twelve planned sessions for these children.

Before the beginning of the first session there had been an unusual incident. The majority of the facilitators were participating for the first time. They had completed their training, and it was the first time they would be working with children in expressive sandwork. A number of experienced facilitators were standing by to offer assistance wherever it might be needed. The group room had been prepared, the sandtrays were set up on tables along the walls, the sand was dampened a little, and the play figures were laid out in the middle of the room, carefully sorted by category so that the children could quickly find what they were looking for. In a moment, the children – whom the facilitators had not yet seen – would enter the room and be allowed to choose a sandtray, as they had been directed. The facilitators sitting next to the sandtrays would, of course, be selected by the children at the same time. While the facilitators were sitting next to their sandtrays and waiting, a young facilitator pointed out that the tables were far too low. Taller children would not be able to work properly under those conditions, she argued. There was a brief discussion, but nobody else shared her opinion. The consensus, and the more experienced facilitators' emphatic opinion, was that the tables had always had the same correct height and that there was no need to change things in the last minute. But the young facilitator would not be deterred. Insisting that her sandtray really was far too low and that her child may not be able to work properly, she asked to be given a higher table. So, to the resentment of many of those involved, a new table had to be produced and was eventually found. Her table was exchanged and finally had the very height she felt it should have. She was content. The other facilitators were somewhat irritated. The children were waiting impatiently out-side the door. Finally, it was opened and they flocked inside the room. A tall, lanky girl, at least a head and a half taller than all the other children, made straight for the only sandtray with the right height for her physique and looked at her facilitator happily and expectantly.

The session began. After the first few minutes of whispering and darting back and forth, silence began to set in as usual. I observed an eleven-year-old girl who, we project leaders knew, had witnessed the murder of both her parents. She had since lived with her grandmother. Normally, we have only little information about the children's family circumstances. But this girl had already willingly told her story to everyone involved and was almost compulsively looking for new opportunities to tell it again. There were no emotions whatsoever in her accounts, however. Her words sounded mechanical and were more likely to cause bewilderment in her listeners than sympathy or compassion. In such situations, sandwork offers a unique possibility to interrupt this kind of vicious circle that is keeping the individual in a psychological trap. It is interesting to see that sandwork immediately constellates themes pertaining to the available resources, and *not* representations of the initial traumatic event. Indeed, I could see that the girl had depicted a beach, complete with sunshades and deckchairs, a few trees, and the sea in front. She took plenty of time over the little details. When she was finished, she remained sitting in front of her sandtray, lost in thought and looking at the beach in front of her. In the team session, her facilitator told us what the girl had said about the beach. She had said it was a place she had often visited with her parents. The beach made her happy and sad at the same time. The scene had deeply moved the facilitator. The girl had *not* told her the story of the murder. Working in the sand in the security of the group had aroused something in the girl that had been concealed until that point. She had been able to activate a memory from *before* the time of the traumatic experience. She had uncovered a resource and reconnected with her emotions. A real process of mourning and emotional processing of the trauma had thereby begun.

Most of the children were already at work, fully focussed, when I noticed a ten-year-old boy who appeared to find it difficult to engage in the play process. He was looking around, a little lost, as if trying to understand what the other children were doing in their sandtrays. Clearly, no ideas of his own were coming to him. Each time he went to fetch play material from the middle of the room he would watch another child and then take the exact same play figures. Returning to his sandtray, he stood rooted to the spot in front of it and appeared not to know how and where to place the figures in the sand. He glanced around beseechingly, his shoulders heaving and his expression sad and frustrated. One could almost hear him thinking, "How ugly my sandtray is. The whole thing is just stupid!" He looked up at his facilitator as if seeking confirmation and help, lifted his shoulders in a questioning manner, fetched another play figure and, once again, appeared not to know what to do with it. It was hard to watch him. I felt an urge to embrace and to hold him, because it appeared as if the sand-tray was drastically confronting him with an unbearable inner emptiness. Tension was mounting inside him, and I wished that his facilitator would do something to ease the strain. But she did nothing, and I wondered whether she had even perceived his dilemma.

After a while, I saw that the boy had set up a scene which was an exact copy of the scene of another child playing next to him. There were some trees, a house, and a "superman" figure. Every-thing appeared randomly placed. The boy regarded it wearily. Then, all of a sudden, he cleared everything aside with a determined movement. He seemed to have finally had an idea because he returned to his sandtray with a handful of soldiers and knew exactly how to place them. He set up an army, and then more soldiers on a raised platform that he had patiently constructed with wooden blocks. Then he switched positions, went to get more soldiers, and placed these in the sand as well. What a relief it was to see the boy play! The facilitator was relieved as well. She reported later that she had very strongly felt the child's dilemma and his incapacity to fully engage in anything. The feeling had even been physical, like a personal blockade. She had wanted to say something to help the child, but she didn't know what. As the session was nearing the end, the volunteer asked the boy if he wanted to say anything about his sand image. He explained the acts of war and pointed out, "These here are soldiers. And this is a child." The facilitator was shocked to see that amidst the army of soldiers there was a smaller soldier running along – a child. After the session, the boy looked as if a great weight had been lifted from his shoulders. He had found the courage to portray a difficult issue that had to do with his own life. He had been able to communicate that there is a child living in the midst of a battle, unable to live the life a child should be able to live. And he had wanted an adult to witness this injustice.

There were only a few more minutes until the end of the session when I noticed a ten-year-old girl in a miniskirt, with a provocative neckline, thick make-up, and deeply sad eyes hectically rummaging through the play material containers. Apparently, she had something very specific in mind and wasn't finding it. Then she selected two wooden sticks, a piece of paper, a pair of scissors, a pencil, and some glue. She cut a rectangle out of the sheet of paper and started writing on it. Her facilitator, she later told us, was silently hoping for the girl's sake that there would be enough time for her to finish her plan. The girl had now stuck the paper rectangle to the two wooden sticks, and the whole construction had become a placard. "Another five minutes," the group leader announced – as always when the session is drawing to a close, so that the children are not taken by surprise. An audible sigh went through the room, and an air of hasty determination to complete unfinished work filled the space. Particularly during the first sessions, a lot of children find it hard to stop. A number of children had already begun offering explanations about their sand images. Eager whispering began to fill the room, the facilitators' body language signalled undivided attention, and their eyes radiated joy over every word their children bestowed on them. The girl had finally managed to get the miniature placard to stand upright in the sand. The letters on the paper could only be read by the facilitator, because it was in her direction that the placard was facing. I read the words after the session, once all of the children had already left the room: "A place for me and Veronica". Veronica was the volunteer's name. Just one month later, the girl came to the sessions without make-up and provocative clothing and played in a manner that befit her age. And one month later yet again, her teacher reported that the girl's performance at school had improved so much that she was about to finish the year as the top of her class.

Once a session is over and the children have all left, the sand-work facilitators always remain seated in the now silent room, reflecting on details in the sand images and completing their notes. Then they begin to clear up, removing the play figures from the sandtrays with the same care and devotion with which the children had placed them there. The creative process unfolds before their eyes in reverse, buried objects often being discovered and excavated layer by layer, as if the volunteers were archaeologists. Often emotions already felt during the session return, but stronger and more unreservedly. During this process, which each facilitator undertakes alone, but in which everyone involved is yet silently connected, someone in the room will often be moved to tears.

SIXTH CHAPTER

Expressive Sandwork
with Refugee Children in Germany

The group as an alchemical container of transformation

We have already established that expressive sandwork takes place in a group consisting of twelve to fourteen children and as many adults. These dyads formed at the outset remain constant for the duration of the whole project. This arrangement means that every child has access to a personal, intimate reference figure. It also eliminates the risk of inexperienced adults taking action because no adult is ever alone with a child. Thus, during the course of the sessions, every individual is able to build trust in the group and is able to experience a sense of security and freedom at the same time. The group is seen as an alchemical container that needs to be hermetically sealed for the process of psychic transformation to occur. As soon as psychic processes begin to express themselves in the children's play and in the relationship structures, the emotional "temperature" begins to rise, everyone's involvement is intensified, every gesture becomes significant, and every observation important. The subtlest emotions are noted, and every individual is connected and in unconscious energetic interaction with every other individual present. This web of interconnectivity increases from session to session. It is understandable, therefore, that outsiders wishing to "just watch" a sandwork session cannot be allowed in. Constant conditions and a little time are needed for this group atmosphere of heightened inner and outer awareness to set in. When it does, words are replaced by eye contact and gestures, and bodies communicate with each other on an immediate level. Those involved often describe the experience as strenuous, but also as relaxing, stimulating, or even paralysing, very much like the countertransference phenomena in an individual analysis setting. The atmosphere is always perceived as energetically charged because every group is larger than the sum of its parts. Should an outsider nevertheless once be admitted to observe a session, it may well be a lost session for the children, and this becomes apparent in their completed sand images. I have written about this in detail in the chapter "The free and protected space is disturbed".[9] The space and time of a session are like a domain that is separated from daily life, where every action, every thought, and every emotion is assumed in advance to carry significance: although we often don't know the exact meaning of a perceived phenomenon, we follow the assumption that there *is* a meaningful context, which pertains not only to the individual, but always also to the group. This assumption creates an atmosphere that leads facilitators – when they are invited to describe their experience in the group – to use the word *magical*. We shall see in the following what this is related to and what effect it can have. Expressive sandwork was begun in Germany in 2016, a year after the large stream of refugees had reached Europe and almost a million people from war zones had found refuge in Germany.

Jungian child analyst Christiane Lutz writes:

[9] Pattis Zoja, E. *Sandplay Therapy in Vulnerable Communities: A Jungian Approach*, Routledge 2011

The current refugee situation calls for pedagogues and therapists to seriously consider traumatic experiences in children and adolescents, and to find ways and means of processing them. A neurotic attempt to deal with burdening experiences is to suppress fear, insecurity, and homelessness from one's consciousness through aggressive behaviour. This is why aggressive interactions are frequently observed between children and adolescents in refugee accommodation. Because these children often come from very different countries, there are also language barriers. The new language, German, as yet imperfectly spoken and laden with abusive terms of an anal and sexual nature, becomes a questionable means of communication. Social competency is highly restricted.

Refugee children therefore often exclude each other and quickly become unloved outsiders and scapegoats in school. The loneliness they experience becomes a yearning for connectedness. This often increases an idealised attachment to the lost homeland, along with a heightened dependency on family, even if this is not befitting of the children's developmental age. This, in turn, restricts the development of appropriate autonomous impulses, and hinders integration into the new home country. At the same time, many of these adolescents live in permanent fear of being deported. This often affects their willingness to fully engage in new personal contacts and to open up to the different circumstances and values in the new country without prejudice.

The first expressive sandwork project in Germany took place in a home for refugees in Baden-Württemberg in 2017 and presented the method with new challenges. We were able to draw on experience from working with refugee families in Colombia, Palestine, and Ukraine, as well as on experience with the Rohingya people in Kuala Lumpur, Malaysia. These Muslim refugees from Buddhist Myanmar are currently one of the people that is most persecuted and threatened by genocide in the world. The Muslim "host" country had never really accepted them. With an officially illegal status, the adults had no hope of being allowed to work, and the children were not allowed to attend schools. The only lessons the children received were from the Koran school that an imam had organised on his own initiative. The group of fourteen adult facilitators for this Rohingya group, on the other hand, consisted of seven different religious affiliations: Muslims, Hindus, Sikhs, Catholics, Greek-Orthodox Christians, Buddhists, and Daoists. The children and facilitators had no means of verbal communication.

In the home for refugees in Germany, on the other hand, the groups' homogeneity and heterogeneity were exactly reversed. The group of facilitators consisted exclusively of German students of psychology, psychotherapy, and pedagogy, while seven countries with different cultural and religious backgrounds were represented in the group of twelve children between the ages of six and twelve (Iraq, Syria, Afghanistan, Eritrea, Kosovo, Albania, Turkish Kurdistan). The adult facilitators were able to communicate with the children to a certain extent. Some of the children spoke English, others understood German. The situation, therefore, was different, and we wondered what impact it might have on the expressive sandwork setting.

The children came to the sessions from different accommodations, and some of them were moved to other apartments during the project. There were families that had just recently arrived in Germany, and others that had already been here longer, which had a clear effect on their attachment security. Even showing up on time for the sessions' beginnings posed a problem for many of the children. Some came too early, others too late or needed to be picked up. We learned quickly that we could not take our own German punctuality for granted.

Organising the parent meetings ahead of the sessions had been difficult because it required up to six translators. The information pamphlet for the parents had been printed in multiple languages. More parents had initially responded than could actually take part, but none of them appeared for the first parent meeting. We learned that the different ethnic groups in the home for refugees scarcely communicated with each other, and that they were not accustomed to attending a joint meeting. This lack of group cohesion was also reflected in the first session with the children. Almost none of them made use of the opportunity to take possession of their own sandtray and be allowed to build whatever they wanted inside it. What is more, the children appeared not to notice the facilitators or to ignore them intentionally, perhaps for fear of being controlled. One of the facilitators, who understood Kurdish, overheard a child whispering to another, as they entered the room, "What do you think they intend to do with us now?!"

And so, at the beginning of the session, the children huddled on the floor in groups of two, three, or four, separated by country of origin, eyeing the play material and conferring amongst each other in their own languages. This filled the room with an unaccustomed atmosphere. There was chaotic buzzing and whispering, while the facilitators sat somewhat helplessly next to their as yet untouched sandtrays. Our interpretation of the situation, which we discussed together after the session, was that the children were expressing something like, *"What are we supposed to do with all these toys? We just don't understand it. We have to find out what we want to do next."* The individual facilitators were a little unsure of themselves because it was their first project, and the situation had developed so differently than expected, but they understood the children's desire for self-efficacy. Therefore, we confirmed to each other via eye contact that we would not intervene but would first wait and see. Some of the children had found their way to a sandtray and corresponding facilitator and started placing objects in the sand, while others stayed sitting on the floor, playing there. Three girls from Iraq had discovered train tracks and began joining them together. Element for element, the track grew in length until it had become a large circle. A little boy from Albania had found a locomotive and some small wagons, and placed them on the tracks. Having received the girls' consent, he moved the train carefully along the wide circle. All of this took place with great calm and concentration. The Iraqi girls who had built the circle appeared content, and the other children, who were already working in their sandtrays, appeared to notice them only peripherally. In the team discussion after the session, it became apparent that the facilitators had almost all had the same thought. These children have travelled a very long way; they were on a journey, seemingly endless in their subjective experience, full of dangers and un-certainties. Perhaps they were still journeying on the inside and would still take a long time to arrive in their host country.

The adults present perceived the initial feelings of uncertainty, tension, anxiety, and agitation gradually falling away and making way for a sense of heaviness and strong compassion. Seeing the circle formed by the tracks on the floor and the train being moved by the child's hand was a moving moment for everyone, and we silently shared the hope of having come a step closer to under-standing these children's experiences.

Weekly sessions followed. The children attended gladly and worked with dedication and the utmost concentration. Nevertheless, there were often a few children missing, either because their parents had not brought them to the session on time or had pursued other activities at short notice. Facilitators and project leaders felt they needed to recreate the free and protected space from the beginning each time.

By the fourth session, the children had already become accustomed to the procedure. A group facilitator[10] wrote:

---

[10] Susanne Wagner, Stuttgart

Once everyone had arrived and the door to the sandplay room was opened, there was immediate calm – it was really hard to believe. There were eleven children and all of them made straight for their sandtrays and started creating things inside them. The children were able to engage fully in their own processes. There was nobody playing on the floor. Many of the facilitators felt an overall sense of heaviness and depth. The children were able to claim the space they needed, and to reveal themselves. So much of what I experienced moved me, and I perceived the group itself as comforting and supportive.

Another group facilitator[11] describes the further course of events:

It was striking how different the atmosphere could be. There were hours when the children were able to concentrate deeply on their own inner images, and other sessions filled with a restless and tense air. In some children, it was outright palpable that they were still fleeing – finishing their sand images as quickly as they could. Others were unable to find a finishing point and had to be urged to finish their work. The children – the central characters in this project – sometimes wondered about the silent observation and occasional note-taking of their facilitators. But they were able to interpret this appreciative attention as affectionate relatedness more matter-of-factly each time. They engaged in the process with great inner commitment. As an observer, one often had the impression that they understood the significance of their silent actions.

---

[11] Christiane Lutz, Stuttgart

In discussions about the role of the facilitator, the call for engaged emotional perception rather than a judgemental and interpretive attitude is usually central. This means facilitators should be perceptive to atmosphere and states of mind on the one hand, but also to their own countertransference emotions that will inevitably arise. Thorough documentation of the events, both during the process and afterwards, ensures certainty regarding these perceptions – as does the photographic record of the sand images themselves.

Seen as a systemic entity, a number of groups are in constant interaction with each other in expressive sandwork: the group of volunteer facilitators, the group of children, the project leaders, the teams of the different institutions involved, the sponsors, and, last but not least, the branching group of the wider international network. Despite obstacles and crises, all parties involved are invited to help make the groups align with the available resources again and again: both in the individual sessions with the children and at an organisational and institutional level. Non-violent communication is emphasised in all internal and external communication (Marshall B. Rosenberg). In the case of critical comments, the main emphasis is to convey underlying needs. Before and after the sessions, while setting up the room and clearing the material away, there is no small talk between the facilitators. There is also no unrequested commenting on other facilitators' children. If observations were made about another facilitator's child, care is taken to first ask the facilitator if he or she would like to hear them. As a matter of course, the completed sand images are also shown this respectful attitude because they are seen as images of the soul of both parties, that of the child and the facilitator. While the children are working in the sandtray, intense psychological forces can be unleashed in the observing adult because unconscious, often highly explosive content from the children's realm of experience can be brought to the surface. Each facilitator works individually with "his" or "her" child, but, at the same time, each individual is also subject to the collective, emotionally charged atmosphere – and of course influences it in return. To ensure that these group processes are accompanied appropriately, for every group of twelve to fourteen children and their volunteer facilitators, the expressive sandwork setting also calls for two to three group facilitators. These are volunteers who are not assigned a child of their own, so that they can keep an eye on the well-being of the group as a whole. They ensure that each child is content in its creative work and intervene if needed to prevent escalation. Their task is to absorb the atmosphere as a whole and to accompany the group-dynamic processes attentively, like an all-embracing vessel.

Experience has shown that these group facilitators, who are not in a position to react empathically to the actions of individual children, are much more immediately exposed to the effects of unconscious content becoming activated in the room. Therefore, the projections, projective identifications, and somatic reactions they experience within themselves are very intense, and must be processed accordingly. These facilitators act as catalysts for the entire system and also begin the process of psychological digestion of elements.

One group facilitator[12] from a project in Munich describes her experience:

> The role of group facilitator was a new one for me, and I perceived it as a field of tension between structured and free space, between observing, coordinating, identifying needs, and deciding between action and non-action. When interventions were necessary, it was always important to differentiate between protecting, holding back, regulating, providing impulses, and acting in support of the facilitators. All in all, I would describe

---

[12] Gabriele Krause Herrmann, Munich

it as a serving role. Regarding the group processes themselves, it is as if all of the people in the room interact as "one organism," i.e. a visible and palpable, yet subtle structure of relationships, with sub-processes, interdependencies, and specific localisations and manifestations (the dyads). It strikes me as a healthy organism, regulating itself and striving to continue its development.

The impulses for this continued development emanate from the interactions, which also act as catalysts. In my role as a group facilitator during twelve sessions, I saw that even the children often have a regulating effect amongst each other: the older children recognise the order of things surprisingly quickly, and some begin to support it, without this ever having been articulated or asked of them. Almost unnoticeably, this sets a process of harmonisation in motion, which affects the play behaviour of individual children, but also the eye contact, facial expressions, and gestures between children, between facilitators, and within the individual dyads. Clearly, there is a continuous process of regulation within the complex interrelationship of association and dissociation. I was also able to observe the structural complexity of the relationships and roles, and the rapidly changing situations in which each sandwork session takes place. A central aspect is the so-called *containment*. This describes the entirety of subtle, open-ended energies in the process that we as facilitators not only perceive, but also absorb, in order to consciously feel them and resolve them inside ourselves. Furthermore, the containment we want to provide is integrated within the overall setting – represented by a number of people going through similar processes here with us, or in other countries and other continents.

The following are notes from the first and from the twelfth session. They were recorded during or immediately after the sessions, and are given here in their raw form to provide a more immediate impression of the facilitator's state of mind and thought associations.

First session:

The first sandwork session begins. I feel full of excited expectation, and can sense the same feeling from the circle of facilitators.

...before the children arrive: All consultations have been brought to a conclusion, the setting is ready, the facilitators have taken their places next to the sand-trays, the children are awaited. The wait is longer than expected... The project leaders move around the house to "help out" with the organisation. As suspected, things don't go entirely smoothly this first time regarding the children's punctual arrival. There are so many people involved... the mothers, the many contacts for the circle of parents, the sandwork team... and of course the children who are the central characters in all of this... There is an almost meditative silence in the room. I ask myself: what else is happening at the same time in the house... with the mothers... with the children... how are things going? I stand at the open door to the group room and listen for sounds from the hallway outside. I think about my task ahead... this new role with a new work approach, within a new team... I ask myself: where, in fact, is my place in this room? For the moment, at the door – that's for sure. And then? I remain pragmatic; keep breathing and maintain eye contact with the facilitators. This is my first perceived impulse for the "support" I intend to provide in the time ahead.

...the children arrive: A number of dark-skinned children pour into the room, accompanied by E. and L. The children are clearly searching for direction in this wealth of impressions of people, play material, and sandtrays. They look around, but most of them quickly reach for the play material.

Things become a little chaotic – a lot of movement, a high level of noise... I keep breathing, firmly confident that some form of order will emerge. I see a number of little interventions from one of the project leaders in particular, trying to get the children to find "their" sandtray and their place – the children do not appear to perceive the facilitators as reference persons at this point.

...many of the children are soon playing:

Most of them are quickly preoccupied with the large selection of play material and spend a lot of time in the middle of the room with the material containers. Of course there is a lot of communication. A number of children sit down on the floor, exploring the play material and beginning to play right there. Through little interventions, the children (almost all of them) gradually begin to understand how and where they are allowed to play, that we are all here in silence, that they should only work at their own sandtrays, etc.

...Silence and chaos: The perceived commotion increasingly turns to phases of silence. Every now and then something flares up and needs regulating, only to find order once more through further interventions. I believe I see the first signs of a healthy process of self-regulation – individually and collectively – within the group. I feel intense joy and breathe a sigh of relief: most of the children have spontaneously accepted the offer, have fundamentally recognised the order of things and have adjusted astonishingly quickly.

...I feel like a kind of "living question mark" in my role: my eyes sweep across the room, gathering and sorting impressions, perceptions, and snapshots. I have found a spot at a wall from where I can observe everything well. I breathe and access the kind of animated silence inside myself that is also palpable in the room to a certain degree. I relate to E. and L., as the "experienced ones" in this work. Where are they at the moment? What are they doing? Are they observing or having to intervene? What impression do the individual facilitators make? Does anybody need anything? What is each child doing, and where? Where is intervention necessary, and what is able to regulate itself on its own? I feel suspended in a field of tension between observing, perceiving situations, and acting upon them – or not acting. Slowly, I begin intervening with some of the children myself, and watch for signals from the facilitators to see if I can assist in my role in any way. This means I leave "my" position at the wall more and more, and move freely through the room. Through eye contact, gestures, or maybe a light touch, I let some of the children – who are still all strangers to me – know that they should be more quiet or should not disturb the other children, remind them where their "own" sandtray is, etc. I am also driven by the motive not to intervene "too much" by acting prematurely or with the same impulse and at the same time as E. or L. Sometimes I notice myself taking a step forwards, only to step back again immediately.

End of the first session: The children worked right up until the last available moment. The end of the session was signalled by a note on the singing bowl. On the one hand, most of the children appeared "played out", but at the same time they needed reassuring that they would be allowed to come again next week. Compared to the impression of the children's entrance, their departure appeared more calm, ordered, and collective. I was tired.

Since nobody is required to follow a specific pattern of observation, neither to systematically record the play sequences nor to exactly capture the children's body language, the observing adults open up to an unaccustomed and very complex experience. They are obliged to perceive and record the flow of thoughts and emotions without judgement: especially for lay facilitators, it is more important to "go along" with events during the session than to feel pressured to reflect on them at the same time. For well-trained psychotherapists, the one does not preclude the other. They are used to experiencing the moment intuitively and reflecting on it at the same time. The following are the same group facilitator's notes from the twelfth session. Much psychological processing has taken place in the meantime.

Twelfth session:

I find it has proven beneficial not to let all the children into the room at once, but in smaller groups instead. This makes for a quieter beginning to the session in the room. Today, again, the children make straight for the boxes with play material in the centre of the room. Eye contact with their facilitators will often only occur later. All except D.: he enters the room last, a little late, and immediately establishes contact with I., his facilitator, and the play material at the same time. It is an absolute joy to see this.

I feel a sense of calm delight when I see how well the children have grown accustomed to the procedure. The necessary interventions are limited to the "classic" ones, as it were: reining in excessively lively communication at the boxes of material, reminding some of the children of their sandtrays... I sense that the facilitators have taken to their positions in a calm, matter of fact way. I consider what a gift it must be for the children to experience this dependable, attentive presence.

Here is the second group facilitator's[13] summary after the final session of the same project. She addresses the progress made by two children in particular.

Multiple levels of support and resources are visible and palpable. I was able to experience the "free and protected space" and the offer of creative play very tangibly from the beginning. I was moved every time to see the children absorb this special atmosphere – in their play and in their resistance. I find it easy to qualitatively describe the changes I perceived between the first and twelfth sessions. It was wonderful to see how confident the very timid girls became in the later sessions. And how much more settled the "trouble-makers" became. I noticed two boys in particular and will outline their cases here briefly. One of the boys was actually far too young for the project – not even four years old – and possibly developmentally challenged. At least that is how he appeared in the beginning: rhythmic rocking motions, scarcely any eye contact, difficult to speak to, ambivalently running towards the left until he came up against a kind of invisible wall,

---

[13] Lia Reznicek, Munich

confusion, backtracking to the right, etc. He seemed interested only in the other children's sandtrays. Each session, I was able to observe how he would eventually end up at his own sandtray next to his facilitator, how she came to get him each time, how he began to discover colourful glass marbles, and how elated he was when he tossed them in his sandtray for the first time. The joy with which his facilitator witnessed his actions, and which she reflected back at him, were just as moving. His actions in play became more purposeful, but also developed an element of "letting go". The boy used his facilitator as an anchor point and then also developed eye contact with the rest of us. He had arrived, and I perceived his presence.

The other boy was ten years old and often came to the sessions filled with aggression. He much preferred to stay in the centre of the room rather than at his sandtray; he spoke loudly, handed out play material to the other children, taunted some of the other older boys, acted up, and laughed at the sand images of the younger boys. This pattern continued over many sessions and even became more pronounced precisely because the other children gradually became calmer and more focussed. This boy's facilitator always remained focussed on him and tried to engage him with her calm presence. We group facilitators did the same. In the tenth session, the boy expressed to his facilitator that he would like to place the sandtray on the floor. Then he sat on the floor like the little children, played for a long time, made circles of butterflies in the sand, and hummed quietly to himself. It moved me in that moment to finally perceive him as a child. The two last sessions with him did not quite go without interventions, but they were clearly different. For example, his interactions with the other older boys no longer consisted of shoves and pranks, but of offers to play together.

I was very interested to know whether the changes that had been so obvious to me in the room were also apparent in the children's regular environment. The social worker who usually cared for the children confirmed my thoughts exactly: something had grown calmer in the children, it was easier to speak to them, they found it easier to learn, they played differently with each other.

Christiane Lutz summarises her experience of the project:

Expressive sandwork with refugee children confirmed our conviction (which was also repeatedly expressed by C. G. Jung) that therapists become givers as well as receivers in a therapeutic process... Time and again, it became apparent how our humanness is defined by polarities. Traumatic experiences of any kind – distressing events, conflicts, suffering, despair – always also mobilise the polar opposites: vitality, strength, endurance, and a will to survive. Having tentative faith in this pheno- menon at first and, as the work progressed, increasingly believing in it as a matter of fact, permitted everyone involved to remain confident, despite all of the pertur- bation, heartfelt sympathy, and occasional helplessness. Faced with the encountered difficulties of conducting the project as planned, some of the sessions brought us close to the end of our tether. And then there were the feelings of grief, fear, and aggression experienced in countertransference. But at the same time the sand images also kindled hope, and fortified our belief in the self-healing ability of the psyche.

Expressive sandwork demands a high level of responsibility. We encourage past negative experiences to
surface, and are aware that we then have to engage
with them on a deep emotional level and in a positive,
holding manner. The children should not feel threatened
by their own sand creations. Instead they should sense
the dependability of the facilitator and come to rely on
it more and more. Providing all of this without words
is often a Herculean task.

Another project with refugee families in Germany took place in
a home for Yazidi women and children. In 2015, 1,000 Yazidi
women were saved from IS captivity and brought to Baden-
Württemberg in a concerted effort directed by Kurdish psychiatrist
Jan Kizilhan. They received resident status through a special quota
and joined the 150,000 Yazidis already living in Germany. On top
of the post-traumatic stress disorders from which these women
and children already suffered, there now also came the element of
cultural shock. Though they were now in safety, they had to adapt
to an unknown social-cultural environment. Naturally this is the
case for all refugees, to a certain degree, but for the Yazidis,
belonging to a religion older than Islam and with a particularly
strong sense of communal life, the transition is especially
pronounced. Therefore, Yazidi women only go out in public in
groups, or at least in pairs. All available rooms in their refugee
accommodation are used and cared for communally, and there is
no knocking on doors. The Yazidi women have not yet availed
themselves of the offer of individual psychotherapy. Expressive
sandwork has proven beneficial in such situations. We already
experienced in Colombia that collective traumas require more than
just individual treatment. They must also be processed within a
community. Collectively oriented populations are quick to accept
the offer of working in a group. It is as if this is precisely what they

had been waiting for, because they are intimately familiar with the supportive and transformative functions of a group activity. The non-verbal means of expression in sandplay are a further facilitating element.

The potential effect of expressive sandwork in extremely traumatised children is illustrated by an episode with this group of children. The Yazidi children who lived in the refugee accommodation with their mothers were often aggressive in their daily interactions with one another. They also showed little hesitation to humiliate each other, which I ascribed to their captivity at the hands of IS, and the things they must have learned from negative models in those two years. At the same time, one could sense that they came from a cultural context where children were treated with attention and respect, and that they basically displayed secure primary attachment behaviour. Since the Yazidi religion considers the four elements and many animals sacred, it was safe to assume that these children had a good relationship with nature and with their own bodies. In addition, their up-bringing would have been oriented towards the community with an emphasis on morality, and their strong sense of cultural affiliation would have been nourished by a wealth of myths, stories, rituals, and symbolic representations passed down through generations. These stories include the persecution, aggression, and injustice the Yazidis have suffered over the centuries, which were never, however, countered with hate or revenge, but merely with a gradual withdrawal of the population to one mountainous region in the north of Iraq. The pride in having preserved their own traditions and never having renounced their own religion despite massive Islamic onslaughts, plays a central role in these narrations. Thus, the children brought a considerable capacity for resilience to the table, and with it good preconditions for processing even the most severe traumas. They were lively, thirsty for knowledge, very interested in their new surroundings, and already spoke good German.

First example:

A nine-year-old boy, who had been in IS captivity with his mother and a number of his siblings, and whose older brothers had either been killed or had disappeared, had already completed six sessions. As is typical of severely traumatised children, he had only ever played v ery briefly, often only for a few minutes. Nevertheless, his facilitator had the impression that a lot had already become activated inside him. His images showed scenes of war, which deeply affected her. What happened next is something that experienced facilitators are no strangers to. If a child feels the urge to communicate a specific element of past emotional life verbally, he or she will mostly not do so with the assigned facilitator. The setting itself is not conducive to intimate conversations between the two. Children in need of a confidant at any given moment in their process will find such a person in their own surroundings, provided the surroundings are safe. It is common, therefore, that children will confide something important in their teacher, their parents, or a social worker, during or after the sandwork project. And so it was in the case of this boy. His teacher had asked the boy a question in front of the rest of the class, and the boy could not answer it. He burst into tears and cried, "Why am I so dumb, why don't I know anything?" And when his teacher reacted and tried to console him, he sobbed on, "Am I so stupid because I have seen the things that IS does?" The boy received encouragement from the class, even his fellow students, and his emotions were adequately caught and held. He had dared to express what might have been weighing on him for months. This was a first, giant step towards processing the things that had occurred. It says a lot for his mental stability that he unconsciously chose a situation – his class in school – that would be able to withstand his outburst. Perhaps the same outburst would have led to a less favourable reaction among his mother and siblings, who were suffering the same trauma.

Second example:

S., a tall Yazidi boy with lively, attentive eyes, balances a soccer ball on his foot and then sends it with an expert kick into an arc that lands it on the nape of his neck. He is eleven years old, speaks perfect German and has never missed a football training session. He very much likes going to school, and his teachers praise his thirst for knowledge. Yet, when the other children romp about in the schoolyard during recess, S. sits off in a corner on the ground and gives himself over to his thoughts. His father was murdered by IS. He too, along with his mother, a sister, and a brother, was captured by IS and imprisoned for weeks in a cellar with scarcely any food and only a pitcher of water. Later he was trained as a fighter. When he speaks about the experience, a chilling smile flickers over his face, and listeners feel a lump in their throat. After the failure of a first attempt to escape from the cellar, S. was separated from his brother and has never seen him again. S. and his mother and his sister were saved by a second attempt to flee.

First session

S. approaches his sandtray as the last of the twelve children who are taking part in the project. He hesitates and appears to have no clear idea as t o what he's supposed to be doing here. He's also the oldest of the children in the group. He casts a glance towards his facilitator, and she responds with an encouraging gesture that gets things underway. So, why not play in the sand, as the younger children are doing? S. begins digging in his sandtray and piles the sand up into mounds. The facilitator writes a few words in her notebook. S. then goes to the array of toys set up in the middle of the room, and comes back with a large black rat. He holds it by the tail, dangles it back and forth, and drops it into the sandtray. He then buries the rat, firmly pounds down the sand on top of it, pulls the rat out again, and repeats the same operation several times. The facilitator's pencil skims across her sheet of paper. S. now takes a rubber frog, observes it at length, and then stuffs sand into its open mouth: so much sand it nearly bursts. This is followed by a flurried search for some other something among the toys while all the other children are concentrated on playing in their sandtrays until S. finally finds a Mikado pick-up stick. He returns to his seat without looking at his facilitator and stabs the stick again and again and from all directions into the belly of the frog. His lips grow pursed into a line. Drops of sweat have formed on his forehead along the line of his hair. The silence in the room has grown heavy. S. now buries the frog deeply into the sand, piles more sand on top of it, and presses it all down flat, again and again, with all his strength. The facilitator's hands grip the edge of her chair; her notebook lies next to the sandtray.

Fourth Session

S. has taken wooden blocks and builds a tall, unstable construction. It is three stories tall, could collapse at any moment, and is surmounted by a skull. He glances repeatedly towards his facilitator: Am I allowed to do this? Will it hold? Will it fall?

Over the course of several following sessions, S. repeats such constructions, which at times remain standing, and at others collapse. When they collapse, he patiently rebuilds them.

Seventh Section

S. sets up soldiers, shoots them with an imaginary pistol, and buries them. He then digs a few of them up, gets hospital beds, lays the soldiers down in them, and surrounds them with figures of doctors and nurses. A game in which alternations of shootings, doctors and nurses, and even surgical operations for the wounded continued throughout several subsequent sessions.

Eleventh Section

Today, S. plays a different game. He has chosen a number of soccer players. He builds a soccer field, with goals, referees, two teams and spectators. He beams at the facilitator and she feels a warm wave of emotion. After setting up all the figures with great attention, rearranging them again and again, S. gives her the signal that the soccer match would now begin. Very carefully, so as not to unintentionally knock down any of the figures, he rolls the soccer ball back and forth from one player to the other, the referees run along beside it on the sidelines, the defenders block, the strikers strike, the public cheers. Goal!

Twelfth and Last Session

S. doesn't show up, and sends the message that he's at soccer practice.

SEVENTH CHAPTER

Expressive Sandwork
in Children Homes in Romania

The number of children growing up in children's homes is larger by far in Romania than in any other European country. The children, between six and sixteen years old, whom we encounter today in our expressive sandwork projects are the grandchildren and great-grandchildren of the generation that was outright forced into fecundity by former head of state Nicolae Ceausescu (1918-1989), with his aggressive demographic policies aimed at turning Romania into a global power. Adequate care was a scarce commodity in the large families that the state not only called for, but actually mandated. A great number of children, both in the countryside and in the cities, grew up in squalor. Many girls themselves became pregnant at a very young age. Abortions were illegal, and so the next generation included a great number of children born out of wedlock, who in turn grew up with insufficient physical and psychological care and were accommodated in state-run children's homes. As late as the nineties, the hygienic and pedagogic standards of these homes could by no means be considered humane. The only alternative to these children's homes were foster families. Foster mothers received a minimum of financial support from the state and had to exhibit reliability and mental stability in order to have children placed in their homes. The same did not apply to the foster fathers living in the same households. In today's state-run and private children's homes there are still many children of school age with two or three failed foster family experiences already behind them, involving regular domestic violence and sexual abuse. In addition to this, there are still children in Bucharest today living in groups in the underground canals of the sewage system. Some of these children took part in an expressive sandwork project. It was necessary to carefully go through the available play material ahead of the project, to remove any rats and bats because some of the children would otherwise react in panic.

Many Romanian children suffer from early attachment disorders, because their parents work abroad and they are instead raised by their grandparents, other relatives or even acquaintances, and are largely left to their own devices. When the parents return on holidays, they are not able to establish a proper relationship with their children. The consequence is disappointment, anger, and depression on both sides. The suicide rate among adolescents is high, and aggressive behaviour in lessons and school drop-out rates are on the rise. Many adolescents are faced with a new problem: after their childhood in environments that offer few stimuli, they are outright catapulted into a world filled with omnipresent virtual images and a steady supply of easily accessible addictive substances. They neither have time to develop their inner emotional stability nor is there anybody to show them how to deal with these new impressions. They are quickly caught up in an inescapable maelstrom of passivity and addiction, and an associated spiral of frustration and violence.

Though Romania's economy has been on the rise in the past decades, and though psychological and psychotherapeutic help from state and private quarters has increased, the number of children and adolescents in need of psychological assistance is still huge. It will take further decades and a veritable army of psychotherapists to mitigate the impact of two generations of neglected children. The long-term consequence is adults with problematic social behaviour and, on a collective, political level, a slowing of democratic processes.

With the following example from Romania I would like to highlight how the offer of expressive sandwork cannot be accepted by the child in extreme cases if a minimum of protection and security are not ensured in the child's environment.

Within a group consisting largely of dark-skinned children from the Roma population (of whom there are approximately 600,000 in Romania), D. was a blond, light-skinned, twelve-year-old boy. He was handsome and had a mild expression and good manners. D. had played unenthusiastically for four sessions, conveying indirectly that he was actually bored by the whole thing, although he did persistently seek eye contact with his facilitator. In the fifth session, he stopped playing after half an hour and said that he didn't want to participate anymore, because this game was for little children. His facilitator invited him to speak to her about it, and they left the sandplay room together, as is usual when a child finishes playing in less than the hour of available time. They found a quiet corner in the common room of the children's home and talked. After some hesitation, the boy explained that it wasn't really the sandplay that he no longer felt like. It was the other children whom he couldn't bear any longer. He couldn't stand "those Roma." They were good-for-nothings, thieves, and criminals and were "harming our country." The facilitator let him finish explaining what he meant and why he found it so unbearable to be in the same group as these children. An immense anger began to surface. "That Roma mob, they should all be shot and eradicated like Hitler did with the Jews. They are vermin and ought to be destroyed. If only I was as strong as Hitler, I would show them. I would shoot them all one by one – bang, bang, bang."

The facilitator was shocked and tried to find an answer that respected her own emotional reaction on the one hand, but also acknowledged D.'s right to deposit his hate without fear of retaliation. She said, "What you are saying makes me feel really afraid. It could just as well be me who is eradicated by you one day." The boy immediately shook his hands and said, "No! Not you! You belong to the good ones; I would never kill you! Definitely not!" There were tears in his eyes. The volunteer offered that he could come to the next session and they could talk again in the common room.

The episode was discussed in the team and provoked pain, helplessness, sadness, fear, and obstruction among the facilitators. Indeed, the boy had a kind of exceptional status in the children's home. Unlike most of the other children growing up there, he only lived in the home part of the time, because he did have a family of origin consisting of his mother and stepfather. He was regularly allowed to return to his family, and the home's administration provided no explanation as to whether this depended on his own behaviour or on other factors.

In the team discussion, the idea was born that the boy's fantasies of destruction could be taken seriously and, paradoxically, be understood in a resource-oriented manner. One could ask him how he would find it if all Roma were indeed gone from the face of the earth, what kind of world would that be?

The facilitator chose this direction in their next conversation. She said she had thought a lot about what he had told her last time, and she had tried to imagine a world in which Roma no longer existed. "Just imagine your wish were really true and there weren't a single..." D. didn't even let her finish the sentence. "That's not even possible," he shouted, "that would never work! I can't do that. I'm not that strong! Do you even know how weak I am? I can't even defend myself against S., my stepfather! You know nothing about me."

The facilitator was silent.

"You know absolutely nothing!" And then it burst from him: "Do you think it's easy? It's anything but! S. beat my mother, and not just once. I think he's beat her at least 40 times – she's covered in bruises. He had stopped until a few months ago, but now he's started again and there's nothing I can do! Can you even imagine that? A man two metres tall and weighing 165 kilos, not fat but strong! Do you have any idea what it's like when someone like that lands a punch? He got me twice and almost broke my arm."

"Is your stepfather Romanian or Roma?"

"He's Romanian. He hates the Roma. He fights them in the streets. Once he beat up an entire family, seven people, men, women, and children."

"Could it be that you got at least part of your anger against the Roma from him?"

"Not necessarily, I hate them anyway. The world would be perfect without Roma. But I would never manage to kill them all. That would make me worse than Hitler. And I wouldn't shoot them all at once anyway. They would have to take a test, and if they didn't pass it – bang, I would kill them one by one. By the way, S. is infamous in the whole neighborhood. Everybody knows him and everybody fears him."

"Does he have a job?"

"He's a thug. His job is to beat up people."

It is easy to understand how a paranoid system could have developed inside the boy's psyche under these conditions. And one could observe this system beginning to falter whenever he became aware of his own powerlessness, then strengthening again, then faltering once more when he managed to speak about the core of the whole matter, his violent stepfather. D. lived in a life-threatening environment and feared for his mother. He hadn't communicated these fears to anybody for fear of losing his right to live with his mother. His time in the children's home did not offer him sufficient security because he still had to fear for his mother's life every day. Aside from any form of therapeutic intervention, D. desperately needed to find a safe environment. The four sessions of expressive sandwork had at least enabled him to speak about his situation. If such a child's cry for help goes unheard, leaving the child as a victim, it is very safe to assume that the paranoid defence mechanisms will gradually establish themselves in the child's psyche and dominate his or her life. D.'s rejection of expressive sandwork had been a life-saving necessity in order to receive the type of help he required in that situation. Unfortunately, we were not able to follow up on whether he and his mother had received the vital protection they needed from the competent bodies.

Another example from a different children's home is offered by F., a thirteen-year-old boy who was renowned in the home for his aggression. He had quickly understood that the project could be an interesting experience for him, but when the children were called in for the first session, he absolutely would not leave behind a stick that he carried in his hand like a weapon. Then F. said he didn't want to take part after all, and his expression looked with-drawn and sad. The project leader had seen how desperately he held on to his stick, which he often used to beat other children. She tried to explain that weapons were not necessary in the sandplay room, because everybody had their own space there and there was enough play material for everyone. The boy shook his head. He would not go in there without his stick. The project leader under-stood that she was about to lose this boy for the rest of the project and decided to take a risk. She agreed, "All right, you can take your stick in with you, but please lay it down next to your sandtray and don't use it during the session." The boy did this, and the weapon accompanied him to all of the next sessions without ever creating a disturbance.

Will the group be disturbed by the behaviour of a single child, or not? This is the relevant criterion when project leaders need to decide whether or not to allow an exception.

We can speak, in this respect, of an interaction of the motherly and fatherly principles. While the facilitator's role is rather allowing and affording in nature, initially accepting any form of behaviour a child might show, the group facilitator's role is to ensure compliance with the rules that are there to protect every-one involved. Taking play material out of somebody else's sandtray, laughing at others, teasing others, and purposefully breaking play material, these are behaviours that attempt to break the frame-work of the setting and they must be prevented. There are no guidelines for how this is done. Each group and each culture has different mechanisms and capacities for self-regulation.

Sometimes it only takes a team discussion, where the facilitators can express their concerns, fear, insecurities, or aggression, and the agitated atmosphere of the previous session will not repeat itself. In fifteen years of expressive sandwork in eight countries, no child has ever had to be excluded from a project for disruptive behaviour. I assume this has to do with the physical sense of security, perceived in the deepest layers of one's personality, which is conveyed by such a large, supportive group. Even the most disturbed children or those with psychopathic tendencies no longer really have an enemy, or someone who needs to be conquered, when they enter a sandplay session. Everything a child needs is available in abundance: play, security, an offer of relationship. Being together or being alone, one is always able to choose what one needs in a given moment. This alone has a calming effect on even the most injured psyche.

Another difficult situation occurred in a home for orphaned children. A twelve-year-old boy was used to being the leader, and the educators had a hard time preventing him from tyrannising and extorting the other children. Even within the sandplay group, working away in silence, it was plain to see that Z. was able to control the rest of the group with just a glance. He completed his own sand image after forty minutes. Z. glanced around the room, and the other eight children obediently ended their playing. Much to the astonishment of the adult facilitators, all the children got up and left the room. The facilitators felt sure that the other children would have liked to finish playing but that the boy had forbidden it. In the following team discussion, the decision was reached not to intervene. Instead the team would wait and see how the dynamic developed further. The second session already appeared to be heading for the same situation, but two of the children were so engrossed in their play that they just didn't notice the boy's commanding, threatening glance, and kept playing peacefully. His power over the group had suffered a first blow. And so it continued session after session. The children cared less and less about his commands and continued playing even after the "boss" had left the room. Despite this loss of power, the boy took part in all the sessions. Unlike the other children, who had made great progress in regulating their emotions, the educators had not noticed any dramatic change in behaviour in the boy. Some of the educators had, however, observed that he had developed a new fascination for little babies. He was exceptionally gentle with them and had recently asked if he could occasionally spend some time in the baby ward. We can assume that the boy had discovered that babies and little children didn't frighten him, that observing their simple existence allowed him to regress positively to a carefree childhood that he himself had never experienced because he, the child of drug addicted parents, had grown up on the streets.

The following are two further short examples of expressive sandwork in children's homes in Romania. The first case pertains to a ten-year-old girl with eating disorders and psychosomatic symptoms and the second to one of countless children whose behavioural problems mask an urge to be seen and appreciated.

These two process descriptions focus on the relationship with the facilitator and on the facilitator's thoughts and emotions. They are intended to show that self-regulation of the psyche is always based on relationship and that the result is always a transformation of both sides involved.

The body is on strike[14]

"Her fingers and wrists are so thin," thinks the volunteer to her-self, as C. begins to play in the sandbox. "Her hands could just fall off those skinny little arms." C. is underweight at age ten, and her dark eyes show no joy in their expression.

"In and out of hospital," explains the foster mother, shrugging her shoulders as if to say: everything has been done, but now even the doctors are tired.

"First there was intestinal irritation, then the ulcer and almost constant inflammation. You can just see the girl getting thinner and thinner. Of course she is. How can she eat with all that pain in her stomach, the poor thing?"

The children around her jump and laugh loudly. C. never wants to sit with them at the lunch table. She sits apart, writing her homework slowly, too slowly. There is a serious risk of impaired growth.

"How can she eat with all that pain?" This phrase sticks in the volunteer's mind.

C.'s mother left her when she was six. She doesn't know why. Nor does she know whether her mother went to Italy or to Spain for work, whether she lives on the streets, or whether she has already had other children. C. had asked a lot about her mother in the beginning, but then she stopped. She decided to wait.

"She is waiting for her mother and she is waiting to grow," thinks the volunteer. "Because growing requires a mother to watch proudly over her child." The volunteer feels a knot in her stomach.

Since sandwork has started, C. plays quietly among the other children, so discreet one could easily forget she was there. Once this actually happened. After all the children had left the room and the team meeting began, C. was still playing unnoticed in her sandtray.

---

[14] Case report provided by Sandwork trainer Julia Feordeanu

She plays with little dolls and makes picnics for them: chooses little plates of similar colours, puts bread loaves on a red table cloth, pours sand in miniature pots and places them on the table.

Her case is discussed in the team meetings. A child who scarcely eats but plays "eating" for session after session? Is this doing her any good? Could it even be harmful? Starving not only at the real table but doing the same in the miniature world as well? On the other hand, her foster mother reports that C. is more relaxed and that she is sleeping better. Maybe sandwork is helping her to better cope with her next hospitalisation?

One month after the end of the project:

The psychologists and volunteers ask teachers and foster parents for feedback on all of the children who were involved in the project.

C.'s foster mother cannot wait to speak. "Do you know what happened? One day, C. came home from school and said, 'From now on I am going to eat with all the other children.' And she has! Her weight is improving each week!"

A thought appeared in the volunteer's mind: "C.'s mother, wherever she may be, can be proud of her, because her little daughter has decided to give life a try."

Who am I?

The boy was born without a birth certificate. Without any legal evidence as to his existence whatsoever. He was the ninth or tenth child born by a woman with severe mental problems and no home or address. Fortunately, the baby's aunt had a job at an orphanage and was able to take him with her to work. T. grew up in the orphanage together with many other children.

"T. is a hyperactive child and can be quite nasty. Something should be done about his aggression," said the teacher.

"What can you do about a child's aggression?" wondered the volunteer, while observing T. play during the first session. Violence and chaos appear to leap out of the sandtray. One scene of war follows another. War, war, and more war. He would shout, "the strongest will win, the others are losers!"

The volunteer can't help but imagine T. as an adult, arrogant, drinking, and bullying others. She loses interest in his play. Her thoughts begin to wander.

Tenth session: The scenes of war kept recurring again and again. The volunteer began to lose hope. By the end of the session, she couldn't have said what exactly T. had played. Surprisingly, after the session, another volunteer who had been sitting next to her came over and said, "I noticed T. playing so quietly today. It was a pleasure to have the two of you close to me."

Eleventh session: The volunteer has gained hope again. Maybe it's true? Maybe T. has changed some of his disruptive behaviour during play? But what is that worth if he doesn't stop taunting others in real life as well? She begins to pay more attention to the scene in the sandtray. "War again, of course!" But then she noticed something different. There is a new feeling to the way he has set up the battle scene, the carefully aligned soldiers, the tanks and the weapons. Just then, as if T. had been reading her thoughts, he explains to her, "You see, this army doesn't fight. These soldiers are exercising. And when they have completed their training, they will compete for this treasure."

"Compete for...", the words echoed in the volunteer's mind, when, quick as a shot, T. looked her straight in the eyes and asked, "What is your name?" Her voice faltered a little as she replied, "My name is G." "G.," T. smiled proudly and continued with his play, talking to her as if she were the child. "You see this treasure? This treasure's name is "G." and all of these soldiers are going to compete for it. And I tell you, they will succeed in getting it!"

G., hearing her own name pronounced in this way by T., the child whose birth had gone all but unwitnessed, can't help but feel that she herself has received a name for the first time.

One month after the project: T.'s behaviour had changed. He is more concentrated, calmer, does better at school, and his social skills have improved.

Who is helping whom?

The facilitators' training, which includes a long weekend of solid introduction and the supervision and intervision sessions throughout the course of the project, emphasises a non-judgemental and accepting attitude towards all appearing content. Facilitators are obliged to direct their attention in two directions simultaneously, to the outside and inside. The outside refers to the playing child and its individual manner of using the miniatures and the sand, the child's play sequences and narratives (should such narratives become clear), the child's posture, facial expression, and moods, and its attempts to establish (or evade) eye contact and relationship in general. The inside, on the other hand, refers to the facilitators' observation of their own countertransference reactions, their changing mental states, surfacing emotions, thoughts, and physical sensations. All these should be written down to ensure that this flow of images, sensations, and perceptions can indeed become conscious. This dual attention is also apparent in the manner of recording itself, either during the sessions, provided the facilitator feels this does not distract the child, or afterwards.

Usually, it is only while going through these notes at a later date that we realise how closely the play content and our own thoughts and inner state of mind were related. This non-judgemental perception of our own inner processes is just as informative as observing the symbolic processes and portrayed narratives in play.

I have always been impressed by how fast lay facilitators learn to use a relatively complicated psychoanalytic instrument like the observation of countertransference reactions and projective identifications. It boosts their vitality and motivation and enables a considerable amount of self-reflection.

It is not unusual for a facilitator to discover remarkable parallels between his or her own childhood biography and the accompanied child's current situation. Or even parallels between both current situations. An example for this phenomenon is presented by the sandplay process of a ten-year-old Romanian girl, whose mother had cancer. Session after session, the child's sand images showed representations of the hospital, the chemotherapy, separation, and death. The facilitator's resilience was severely put to the test each session because she herself was caring for her aunt at the time, who was also terminally ill with cancer. She felt a great sense of fear before each session and worried that she wouldn't be able to bear what the girl would represent in the sand. The presence of the group, who were aware of her situation, was somewhat of a support. During the sessions themselves, the volunteer was impressed with which courage the girl was able to portray her mother's illness. The images repeatedly showed a female figure lying on a rectangular shape, which could have been a sickbed (she was once attached to a machine) or a grave, and she was always enveloped by a wreath of flowers and butterflies, protected, and also appearing to be the centre of a ceremony. These sand images were colourful and radiated vitality on the one hand. On the other hand, they almost crushed the observer with a sense of heaviness and breathlessness. In the second to last session, the mother's face filled the entire image. Her hair was made of grass and flowers, as if she were a goddess of fertility at a harvest feast. The two dark glass marbles representing her eyes were of two different colours. One eye shone blue, and the other green, which gave the face a particular almost unearthly expressiveness. From her ears hung ripe red apples and her mouth expressed deep satisfaction. There was no sadness in this face, it was a picture of natural serenity. The entire sandplay process appeared to be an act of saying goodbye, an examination of the threatening and promising sides of life – and its intensity had taken the facilitator close to her limits.

The following are some of the notes she took after the sessions had finished.

> The emotional impact was very strong in all of the sessions – overwhelming, tormenting. I felt frightened for at least two thirds of the sessions because my own problems from that period were reflected in the girl's sand images (my aunt was dying of cancer). At one point, I felt I couldn't continue the process – it felt too difficult to carry. I often dreaded the approaching day of the next session, and wondered, "What new problem is she going to unearth in me?" I started to take things very personally. When she went to get miniatures for her sandtray, there were many times that I wrote in my notes, "What if she were to bring a certain object now?" And, sure enough, she would bring back that very object more than once. These coincidences triggered multiple contradictory states inside me, joy, happiness, amazement, terror, even satisfaction.

> Sometimes I could hardly hold back from crying. So great was the similarity of her sand image with my own personal problem. Physically, I often felt an immense sensation of heaviness. I remember one time in particular when she fetched stones of many different sizes and filled the sandtray with them. I often had the impression that the girl's process was a very conscious one. There was always order in the sandtray and beauty but also clear opposites (good and bad), dangers, loss,

and sadness. It all appeared intelligent, made clear sense – and was inescapable.

Since I had a great deal of emotional difficulty with this process, I must admit I was relieved when it was over.

The following are descriptions by three children from Romania, who were asked three months after the close of the project what significance their experiences had had for them.

Twelve-year-old boy:
I came to play in the sand. I had a good feeling because there was a lot of silence and everyone was preoccupied with doing the same thing. I realised that when you are in a place like this, where there is silence and you have someone who "helps" you, you can do whatever you want. If you remember, I created a lot of things in the sand.
I liked the fact that I didn't have to do anything specific, but was allowed to do whatever crossed my mind. I was sent home to my mother during that time, but even if unpleasant things happened at home, I knew that I would be able to return to the centre to play in sand, and this thought comforted me.

Sixteen-year-old girl who had been an outsider at school, but went from being last in her class to second best in only eight months:
The lady who was with me wasn't a teacher, for sure. She was different. She accepted me the way I was. She didn't scold me; she didn't make me feel guilty. I think she cared about me, even if she didn't tell me. I felt I was being met with love. As a matter of fact, all the adults

there were different. I think it was hard for them to pay attention to us all the time. That's hard work. I also think they studied a lot. They knew a lot of things. I met other children there who had the same problems as me. They were shy, afraid of making mistakes, and afraid to speak. I used to be shy and quiet. There it felt as if we had known each other since forever. I liked it. I realised I am not the only shy person in the world. I am not like that anymore. I don't feel nervous every time I have to speak. I am able to talk and have relationships with other children. People think of me as a normal person, not a strange one. But the thing I like best is that I am not afraid of making mistakes anymore. Only now have I realised that you can also learn from mistakes. I liked it. I would like to know whom I owe a debt of gratitude for taking me into this project. There must be a boss, and I am sure he is a good boss. I will not forget this project, and when I grow up I will volunteer some-where as well. This project is like a dove in my soul.

Twelve-year-old boy:
I felt good during this project. I liked playing in the sand, playing the way I want to, anything I wanted to. It was fun. At first I didn't have enough time, then I became tired. I didn't want to come any more, but then I managed to do what I wanted in a given time. This project calmed me down. I am not as hectic and rushed as before. I found everything I wanted in the boxes with toys. I would compare this project to a golden crown.

EIGHTH CHAPTER

Expressive Sandwork in the War Zone in Ukraine

Kiev, April 2018

"We will win!" said Boris, the young taxi driver, emphasising each word as he navigated his Mercedes through congested traffic between the airport of Borispol and the city centre of Kiev. A little surprised at how quickly our conversation had moved from the booming Ukrainian folklore music groups to the topic of war, I did not immediately respond. Seeking my eyes in the rear-view mirror, he continued with a touch of forcefulness in his voice. "And do you know why? There are two reasons. First, because we produce our own weapons. We are not dependent on arms trade of any kind. Ukraine produces its own tanks and fighter jets. And second, we are simply more intelligent than them over there." A moment of silence followed, as the joins of motorway segments bumped regularly beneath our seats. A giant stainless steel female figure, the 102-metre-high *Rodina Mat* or "Motherland" – sword and shield held high in her arms – approached on our right-hand side, acquired her maximum dramatic effect of socialist rhetoric in profile, and then passed graciously by, only to disappear behind bright birch forests in the next long-drawn curve to the left.

"Were you at the front in Donbass, yourself?"

"No, but I would go. I have two small children and I would fight for them if I must."

I am making my way to the border area in eastern Ukraine, from where 1.3 million people have fled since 2015. Vlad, a psychologist who has introduced sandwork in Ukraine and coordinates the projects in the Eastern cities, accompanies me in the night train from Kiev to Sloviansk.

The train is fully booked and packed with people. The journey lasts sixteen hours and leads through vast expanses of uncultivated land and forests, interspersed with coal mines and bleak barrack settlements. The final stop is Sloviansk, a small city of about a hundred thousand inhabitants which was taken by the "separatists" just four years ago, in April 2014, and held for three months. A majority of the inhabitants left the city. Two schools and a kindergarten were bombed and flattened. We see bullet holes on buildings. At the same time, the inhabitants have started a concerted effort to beautify their city. Freshly painted facades on a number of one-storied houses offer a cheerful counterpoint to the rows of dilapidated Soviet-style apartment blocks. Apple trees and plum trees blossom in the little front yards. Standing there in radiant white, they look like giant bridal bouquets and give the city a very festive air that is deeply touching. Are people trying to forget the war by any means possible?

For about a year now, the international media has spoken of a "forgotten war" in Ukraine, although soldiers still die there every day in the border areas of the newly declared republics of Donetsk and Luhansk, and although nobody can leave the narrow trails between the villages because the fields and forests are strewn with mines. Once a term like "a forgotten war" has been uttered in journalism, it becomes a self-fulfilling prophecy. Who laid those mines? Nobody knows. Did the Ukrainian army lay mines in their own homeland? Did the "separatists" lay mines in the region of their Russian-speaking ancestors? Nobody knows. I repeatedly hear the words "Njazin, njazin informatia!" spoken in Russian and in an angered tone, in the people's narrative flow. There is no information for the civilian population. The inhabitants point with a sweeping gesture towards the horizon, where the explosions could be seen night after night. There is a note of concern in their accounts that listeners might not quite believe them; that they might believe it was only half as bad; that the whole world might think the war in Syria is always much worse. The people here also lack information about the war's psychological consequences. At the beginning of 2018, UNICEF handed out brochures describing and illustrating the symptoms of post-traumatic stress disorders in children.

Ludmilla, who runs the local kindergarten, reports of parents bringing pre-school-aged children to the psychological counselling service and asking if anything could be done for their handicap. They were "born dumb." Ludmilla points out that sixty percent of children in the war zone, according to statistics of the local polyclinic, exhibit a developmental delay, yet the children's parents and relatives are completely oblivious to any connection with the war. Because the adults themselves would like to forget the month-long bombardments, explosions, shootings, lootings, acts of violence of every kind, and their escape and constant fear, they have no inner readiness to even begin to imagine the shock their infants and young children must have suffered. The conventional wisdom is that the little ones won't have really realised what was going on. Paradoxically, it is easier for the psychological equilibrium of a traumatised adult to accept that a child is born handicapped than to confront the fact that traumas of war have a long-term impact on children's development. If this is suggested to parents as a fact, anger and pain erupts all the more forcefully and they awake from an apathy into which they had fallen for months. And so the population is trapped not only in a concrete borderland where it is threatened with mortal danger from both sides, but also in a psychological no-man's land where relationships no longer function. A crying child is no longer consoled.

But defense mechanisms always also have a protective function and must not be forcefully penetrated through psychological intervention without assistance also being guaranteed. Expressive sandwork offers just such an assistance. Of the 84 children who took part in expressive sandwork in Sloviansk, 85% showed positive behavioural changes, according to their parents.

The following is the example of a five-year-old child in Popasnaja. When T. was three and a half years old, her family's house was hit by a mortar bomb. Her family survived the attack, but T. subsequently lost all of her hair. She also suffered from an intense fear of abandonment, which didn't improve and made enrolment in school unthinkable. Her hair, eye lashes, and eye brows did not grow back. At the beginning of the sandplay project, which would take place without the parents, T. could not be encouraged to join the group. This changed in the fourth session, when the facilitator offered to hold T. in her arms while she played. In this first session for T., she observed the other, older, children for a long time. Even the loudest and most conspicuous among them were silently, almost reverently concentrated in their work. Then T. reached for the sand herself and a big heart formed under her little hands. A joyful look from the girl to her facilitator and a smile on both of their faces constituted the beginning of a psychic healing process. After four weekly sandplay sessions, darker spots began to show on T.'s bare head. Her hair had begun to grow again. For the parents, this was nothing short of a miracle. Is there a clinical explanation? It is safe to assume that the child's fears were adequately met: the project leader had found a good balance between encouraging the girl and granting her space, and had won the girl's trust. The decisive factor, however, had been the child's holistic, non-verbal, and therefore age-appropriate, experience of self-efficacy. Resilience can be defined as reacting actively to an adverse experience. Being able to create an inner world from scratch in a sandtray gives children the most valuable experience of self-efficacy possible. The fragmented inner world is reassembled in a new way, and this has a direct and visible effect on the autonomic nervous system (children sleep better, for example) and on somatic functions. Even if no word is spoken during sandplay, mentalisation processes are constantly occurring. Children can observe themselves from a distance and reflect on their own emotional experience as if through a wide-angle lens. Reflection in young children occurs in the form of "as if" games. These are models for experiencing the world and interacting with it, which provide children orientation and something to draw themselves forward along like a well anchored rope.

X., a group leader from the counselling service in Popasnaja tells of an eight-year old boy, A., who had no better ideas during his first sessions than to disturb all the other children. He repeatedly overstepped the few rules in sandplay that are designed to protect the setting: he threw sand out of the sandtray, took other children's play material, and commented loudly and rudely on their sand images. X. had tried everything and didn't know what else she could do in her role as group facilitator. There was a real risk that a single child could jeopardise the entire project. A. lived with his grandmother, who was very strict with him. His mother had moved away, and he almost never saw his father. In his first sandplay session, A. placed a house in the middle of the sandtray, added a few trees around it, and then placed the figure of a little child on the roof of the house, so that it looked as if it were about to fall off. Then A., almost randomly, fetched a smurf figure with outstretched arms and placed it in the sand next to the house. It looked as if the smurf could catch the child if it should fall. His facilitator was moved by this scene. We understood the image to show that the boy was in great danger of being harmed by his own trans-gressions but that he had also clearly understood that help was available. When A. continued to disturb the other children, X. took him into another room before the fourth session and spoke with him for a long time. Among other things, she said: "A., I see you.

You really don't have to do all these things that disturb us. You are important to us just as you are. Do you understand? We adults, we *see* you." A. looked at her and tears started to well up in his eyes. "But my grandmother doesn't see me."

After this talk, A. became calmer and played quietly in his sandtray. The great success of this story was that his grandmother later came to the counselling service to ask for help. A. is one of the many children who were given another chance at just the right moment through sandplay. The little smurf figure in his sand image represented his capacity for psychic self-regulation, which had become activated. What is more, and this is something that sandplay facilitators witness over and over again, the positive effect also extended to the child's environment.

References

Bowlby, J. (1969). *Attachment.* Attachment and Loss (vol. 1). New York: Basic Books.

Chodorow, J. (1991). Dance Therapy and Depth Psychology: The Moving Imagination. Hove, Routledge.

Hillman, J. (2006). *City & Soul* (R. J. Leaver, Ed.). Putnam, CT: Spring Publications.

Jung, C.G. *Collected Works, Psychological Types,* Vol. 6, Princeton University Press, Bollingen Series XX. par. 757.

Jung, C.G. *Collected Works, Psychology and Alchemy*, Vol. 12, Princeton University Press, Bollingen Series XX.

Kalff, D. M. (1960) Sandplay, a Psychotherapeutic Approach to the Psyche. Temenos Press 2004.

Marshall B. Rosenberg, https://www.cnvc.org.

Neumann, E. (2014). *The Origins and History of Consciousness* (R. F. Hull, Trans.). Princeton: Princeton University Press.

Panksepp, J. (1998) Affective Neuroscience, *The Foundations of Human and Animal Emotions*, Oxford Press.

Panksepp J. & Biven L. (2012) *The Archeology of Mind, Neuro-evolutionary Origins of Human Emotions*, W.W. Norton.

Pattis Zoja, E. (Ed.). (2004). *Sandplay Therapy: Treatment of Psycho-pathologies*. Einsiedeln: Daimon Verlag.

Pattis Zoja, E. (2011). *Sandplay Therapy in Vulnerable Communities: A Jungian Approach*. London: Routledge.

Spitz, R. (1965). *The First Year of Life: a Psychoanalytic Study of Normal and Deviant Development of Object Relations*. International Universities Press.

Stern, D. N. (2004). *The Present Moment in Psychotherapy and Everyday Life*. W.W. Norton.

Stern, D. N. (1990), *Diary of a Baby, What Your Child Sees, Feels and Experiences*, Basic Books.

Stifter Adelbert (1867) Mein Leben: Aus den Nachlassblättern, Kap. 1, Projekt Gutenberg (http://gutenberg.spiegel.de/buch/mein-leben-204/1)

Winnicott, D.W. *Playing and Reality*, Routledge Classic Edition, (1971).